Chinese Medicine Explained

Chinese Medicine Overview, Theories, Philosophies, History, Western Medicine Comparison, Acupuncture, Herbal Medicines, Methods, Patterns of Disharmony and Much More!

By Frederick Earlstein

Copyrights and Trademarks

All rights reserved. No part of this book may be reproduced or transformed in any form or by any means, graphic, electronic, or mechanical, including photocopying, recording, taping, or by any information storage retrieval system, without the written permission of the author.

This publication is Copyright ©2018 NRB Publishing, an imprint. Nevada. All products, graphics, publications, software and services mentioned and recommended in this publication are protected by trademarks. In such instance, all trademarks & copyright belong to the respective owners. For information consult www.NRBpublishing.com

Disclaimer and Legal Notice

This product is not legal, medical, or accounting advice and should not be interpreted in that manner. You need to do your own due-diligence to determine if the content of this product is right for you. While every attempt has been made to verify the information shared in this publication, neither the author, neither publisher, nor the affiliates assume any responsibility for errors, omissions or contrary interpretation of the subject matter herein. Any perceived slights to any specific person(s) or organization(s) are purely unintentional.

We have no control over the nature, content and availability of the web sites listed in this book. The inclusion of any web site links does not necessarily imply a recommendation or endorse the views expressed within them. We take no responsibility for, and will not be liable for, the websites being temporarily unavailable or being removed from the internet.

The accuracy and completeness of information provided herein and opinions stated herein are not guaranteed or warranted to produce any particular results, and the advice and strategies, contained herein may not be suitable for every individual. Neither the author nor the publisher shall be liable for any loss incurred as a consequence of the use and application, directly or indirectly, of any information presented in this work. This publication is designed to provide information in regard to the subject matter covered.

Neither the author nor the publisher assume any responsibility for any errors or omissions, nor do they represent or warrant that the ideas, information, actions, plans, suggestions contained in this book is in all cases accurate. It is the reader's responsibility to find advice before putting anything written in this book into practice. The information in this book is not intended to serve as legal, medical, or accounting advice.

Foreword

Traditional Chinese Medicine has been around for the last 3,000 years! This is a practice that is as old as time. It is an ancient medical system that arises from literate scholars back in the day, and is a living tradition that has been carried for generations especially in the Orient or the East. Chinese Medicine is a well – structured system that has a solid theoretical basis and framework. It is an integral guide in understanding and healing various human diseases, and it's something that has been at the forefront of the health care in the East particularly in China and many Asian countries such as Japan, Singapore, and Vietnam etc. Western medicine is now catching up and integrating this medical system in North American and European countries.

Traditional Chinese Medicine has ever since been viewed as the body's intimate relation to its natural surroundings, and through this relationship, it has become an essential factor in understanding the process of an individual's health. This book will teach you the basic theories of Chinese Medicine, the fundamentals, herbal medicines, acupuncture, and how the system can be applied and act as an aid to the many forms of diseases nowadays. This book will guide you on how this ancient system has stand the test of time and why it is now being practiced more than ever today.

Table of Contents

Chapter One: Introduction to Traditional Chinese Medicine (TCM) 9

Chapter Two: A Brief History of Traditional Chinese Medicine 13

    Ancient Days of the Chinese Medicine (2nd - 1st Century B.C.) 14

    Han Dynasty (200 BC – 200 AD) 15

    Tang Dynasty (618 - 907 A.D.) 17

    Ming Dynasty (1368 - 1644) 19

    Qing Dynasty (1644 – 1911) 21

Chapter Three: Comparison of Traditional Chinese Medicine and Western Medicine 23

    Western Medicine vs. Traditional Chinese Medicine 24

Chapter Four: Basic Theories of TCM: The Yin - Yang Theory 31

    The Yin – Yang Theory 33

    The 4 Fundamental Characteristics of Yin – Yang Theory 34

        Opposition 34

        Interdependence 36

        Interdivisibility and Relativity 37

        Inter – consuming – supporting 38

Intertransformation 38

Yin –Yang Theory Application to Chinese Medicine 39

Chapter Five: Basic Theories of TCM: The Five Phase Theory 41

The 5 Phase Theory and Its Body Correspondences 42

Endangering Cycle 44

Controlling Cycle 45

Application in Chinese Medicine 46

The Use of 5 Phase Theory in Diagnosing Symptoms 50

Five Phases Applied in Therapeutics 50

Chapter Six: Chinese Medicine and Chronic Diseases 53

TCM and Chronic Diseases 54

TCM and Organ Diseases 57

Emotional Instability 59

Diagnosis of Organ Diseases 61

Chapter Seven: Patterns of Disharmony 63

The 8 Yin and Yang Pathologies Diagram 64

Example of Patterns of Disharmony 69

Chapter Eight: Acupuncture 71

Brief History of Acupuncture's Development 72

Traditional Chinese Medicine 75

5 Elements or Classical Acupuncture 75

Japanese Style Acupuncture (Matsumoto) 76

Korean Style Acupuncture 77

Vietnamese Style Acupuncture 77

Classical Balance Method 77

French – Style Acupuncture 78

Significant Researches on Acupuncture 78

How to Receive Acupuncture 81

Chapter Nine: Traditional Chinese Medicine and Cancer ... 85

TCM's Holistic Approach to Cancer 86

Chapter Ten: Chinese Herbal Medicine 91

Brief History of Chinese Herbal Medicine 92

Classification of Chinese Herbs 96

Chinese Herbs vs. Synthetic Drugs 100

Preparation of Chinese Herbal Medicine 103

Types of Herbal Administration 107

Important Basic Concepts to Remember in Traditional Chinese Medicine 111

Important Concepts 112

Conclusion 120

Photo Credits 123

References 125

Chapter One: Introduction to Traditional Chinese Medicine (TCM)

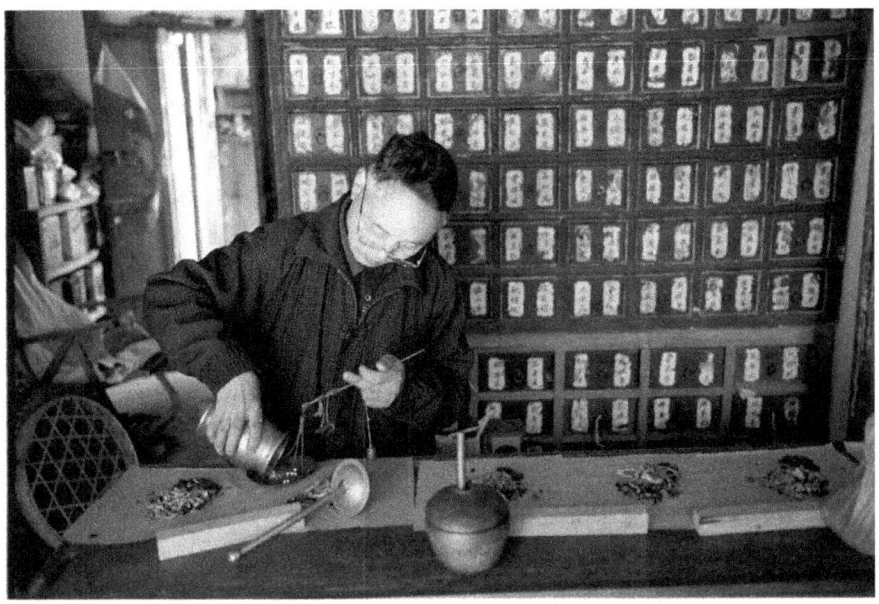

Chinese Medicine is a medical system developed in China thousands of years ago. It has many complementary and alternative features that cannot be replicated in today's modern medicine even with the combination of advanced technologies. TCM's fundamentals are based from abstract theories like the yin and the yang as well as the 5 elements. It is a rational medical system that can be used not just in treatment but also in diagnosis, prognosis and even prevention of certain diseases. It can be an alternative method to treat all kinds of diseases that people encounter today.

The ancient knowledge of this medical system has been systematically passed down by word of mouth and also through a textbook dating back to the 800 to 200 B.C. called "The Yellow Emperor's Internal Medicine" – this textbook is still being used among modern TCM practitioners today. The practice has been continuously developing over the years, and it's serves as an essential pillar in China's health system up until today. (More on this as we cover the next chapter which talks about the brief of history of Traditional Chinese Medicine).

In the ancient days, disease is understood as the human body's deviation from natural conditions and it is something that also corresponds with the changes in one's natural surroundings. In Traditional Chinese Medicine, illnesses are usually caused by the ever changing surrounding around us, it is caused by various and fluctuating conditions such as the cold, heat, dampness, wind etc. all the while, and the body's internal functions are grouped according to the perceived relationships that are

Chapter One: Introduction to Traditional Chinese Medicine

systemic. These descriptions point to the groups of related body phenomena wherein when they occur together, they can be treated with interventions like what practitioners of TCM do such as acupuncture, herbal therapy etc.

There are certain theories that should be used as a guide in order to ensure that the practice of TCM methods like acupuncture and herbal medicine is properly applied. You'll learn these basic theories in the upcoming chapters; such theories are the fundamentals of traditional Chinese medicine. Compared to Western medicine that only focuses on the body's structural changes like the alterations in the blood or tissues chemical compositions, Chinese Medicine focuses more on the alterations of the body's functions.

The patient's conditions must be analyzed under this system if you want to see the full therapeutic manifestation and potential of Traditional Chinese Medicine. TCM also complements the Western biomedicine approach which can provide patients with optimal health care results.

Chapter One: Introduction to Traditional Chinese Medicine

Chapter Two: A Brief History of Traditional Chinese Medicine

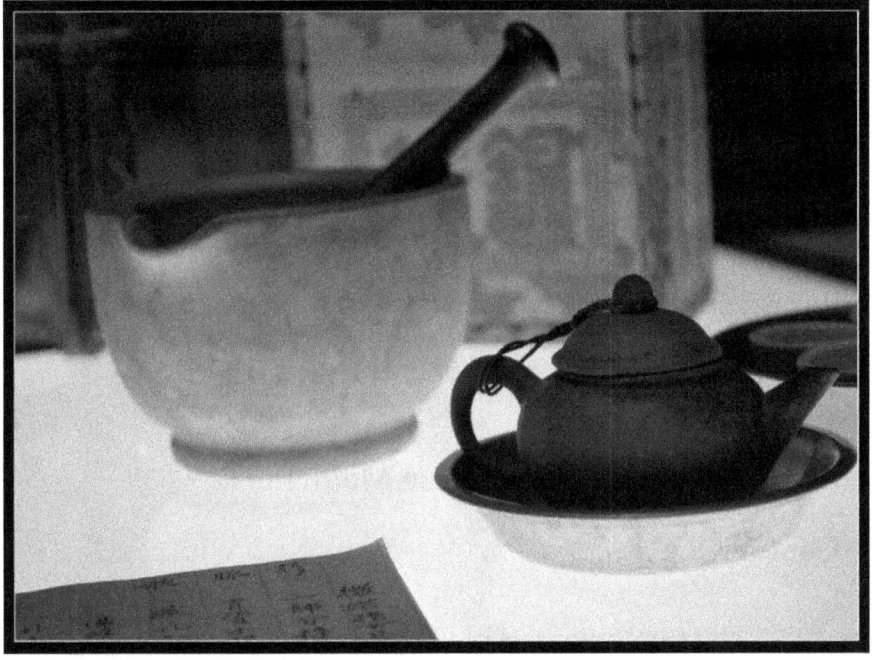

Ancient Chinese inhabitants are the original creators of this alternative medical system. Around 2200 B.C. is where it all began; the ancient orients found different methods of healing illnesses and using it to make the body achieve its optimum performance. The early Chinese, for instance, realized that hot stones can be pressed against certain body parts which could then relieve certain illnesses or muscle pains.

Chapter Two: A Brief History of Traditional Chinese Medicine

They also realized that by using bone needles and pricking it in certain body areas can relieve various body pains - this is how acupuncture was born. Chinese Medicine back then was also used as part of ceremonial magic and other sort of ancient rituals. This chapter will provide you with how TCM came about and its very fascinating history that had been passed on from one dynasty to another up to this generation.

Ancient Days of the Chinese Medicine (2nd - 1st Century B.C.)

The fundamentals of Chinese Medicine in which the system is anchored can be traced back around the publishing of 2 classic books in the 2nd to the 1st century B.C. called *The Yellow Emperor's Internal Medicine* and (the Fire Emperor's).

Classic of Herbal Medicine.

Both of these books lay the basics of this medical system. The theories, principles, philosophy and application

Chapter Two: A Brief History of Traditional Chinese Medicine

including the acupuncture practice and herbal treatment contained within these ancient books largely contributed to how Chinese Medicine is being practiced today. These books were a compilation by many ancient Chinese "medical practitioners," philosophers, and several authors for over a period of time. It has only been attributed to the Yellow and Fire Emperor because it's a tradition back then to assign the author of a book to the masters/ teachers that influenced them but technically speaking, it's a collective knowledge.

Han Dynasty (200 BC – 200 AD)

During the Han Dynasty, author Zhang ZhongJing wrote another Chinese Medicine book called *Shanghan Zabinglun* (Discourse on Fevers and Miscellaneous Illnesses). The book discussed the different ways of diagnosing an illness and treatments methods that can be assessed based on the symptoms of various pathological conditions. This is quite significant because during this time, there's no distinction between infectious and non – infectious diseases.

Chapter Two: A Brief History of Traditional Chinese Medicine

Hua Tuo (145 - 208 A.D.)

Hua Tuo became a significant person in the history of Traditional Chinese Medicine because he is an early anesthesiologist. His skill as a surgeon is quite impeccable. His use of anesthesia is something that is unfathomable at the time. Before he begins surgery, he lets his patients take an anesthesia called Mafeisan which is quite similar to cannabis, and it's very helpful as a pain reliever. Unfortunately, most of Hua Tuo's works were lost and gone. His surgical methods also became unpopular due to certain religious/ cultural beliefs. However, he made a contribution by using herbal medicine such as Mafeisan to relieve pain, and he also recommended and devised different physical exercises to his patients to aid in their recovery. He used the 5 animals of the Chinese tradition (bear, monkey, tiger, bird, and deer) for such movements.

Chapter Two: A Brief History of Traditional Chinese Medicine

Lei Xiao (500 A.D.)

Another Chinese Medicine contributor is Lei Xiao who wrote a book called Liu Juanzi Guifang. The book provides information when it comes to treating skin diseases like abscesses and anthrax as well as wounds caused by metal instruments. His book also mentioned Mercury as an alternative for healing some skin conditions.

Tang Dynasty (618 - 907 A.D.)

Tang Dynasty is the era where Chinese Medicine became quite popular and also has been developed with the help of other Asian countries. This is the time when China have already improved and transportation systems where built. The concepts and theories of TCM spread in other countries including Korea, Vietnam, Japan, and India through the Chinese doctors who visited in those countries. They brought back with them different ideas and methods that they later used in developing further the methods of TCM. Korean herbs like ginseng, Bai Fuzi, and Korean pines were introduced; Vietnam introduced the use of vanilla grass, cloves and sappan. Ophthalmology is something that is discovered and developed by Indian and Chinese Buddhist monks. Indian herbs like angelica and ephedra were also brought to China and are now part of the herbal medicine used.

Liu Wansu (1120 - 1200)

Another popular TCM doctor is Liu Wansu. He's the one who emphasized how essential the fire and heat elements are. He often prescribed "cooling herbs" in order to treat diseases caused by such elements. He later founded a school that teaches his methods and was later known as the "School of Cooling."

Zhang CongZheng (1150 - 1228)

Zhang's innovative approach when it comes to diagnosing and treating illnesses is quite significant. He developed the theory of the Six Doors and Three Methods;

Chapter Two: A Brief History of Traditional Chinese Medicine

Th Six Doors pertains to the six influences that can cause a person to become ill, these influences are heat, summer, dampness, wind, col, dryness and fire. While the Three Methods are the therapeutic regimens he used for healing.

Li Gao (1180 - 1251)

This TCM doctor is famous for his theory on how social factors can affect one's body functions. According to him, emotions play an important role when it comes to being ill. Emotions such as anger, sadness, joy, grief, optimism and the likes can basically influence one's Qi (core energy found in a person based on Chinese philosophies), and can cause certain illnesses.

Ming Dynasty (1368 - 1644)

Wu Youxing discovered that there are some diseases that are transferrable but it can be easily cured by herbal medicines. The usual entrance of such diseases is through the nose and mouth, and the severity of such disease highly

Chapter Two: A Brief History of Traditional Chinese Medicine

depends on the amount/ intensity of this external influence as well as the body's resistance. This discovery has some similarities to microbiology in Western medicine, and this marks the first time in TCM history to propose germs and viruses as causes of epidemic illnesses.

Li Shizhen (1518 - 1593)

Considered as one of TCM's greatest contributor particularly in the field of herbal medicine, Shizhen revised the classifications of many drugs. He created guidelines for the collection, preparation, and administration of drugs in his book called *Compendium of Materia Medica*. In his book, he detailed almost 11,000 drug prescriptions. His book is still used as a major reference today not just in TCM but also in botany, therapeutics, and pharmacology.

Chapter Two: A Brief History of Traditional Chinese Medicine

Qing Dynasty (1644 – 1911)

The development of Anatomy was further developed. Wang Qungren was one of the significant doctors of this era; he published a book in 1830 called Errors Corrected from the Forest of Physicians (Yilin Gaicuo). In his book, he discussed the different body organs and the overall structure of the body such as the pancreas, diaphragm, and abdominal aorta to name a few, which is quite unknown to Traditional Chinese Medicine at the time. He demystified some mistaken beliefs like the heart is not the center of thought and memory but the brain.

Around this time, doctors have also developed preventive measures for smallpox using inoculation as a method. The method was not perfect but it acted as a vaccination for smallpox at the time. They let healthy people who have not had smallpox inhale the dry crusts and scales (which had been reduced to fine powder) that came from the skin of a patient who has smallpox.

Chapter Two: A Brief History of Traditional Chinese Medicine

TCM had since made many significant discoveries and have developed more accurate techniques over the years. Today, it's now being infused with Western medicine and acts as a complement in treating various diseases.

Chapter Three: Comparison of Traditional Chinese Medicine and Western Medicine

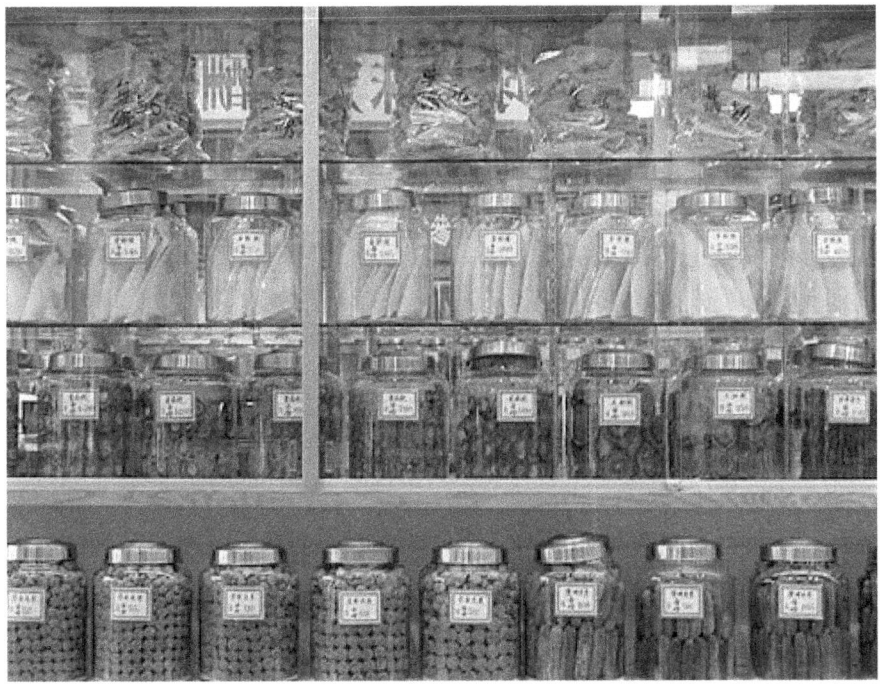

The history of Traditional Chinese Medicine to some extent has some resemblance to that of Western Medicine until around the 18th century. However, as the years go by, both medical systems moved away from the belief that illnesses were caused by supernatural forces but rather it is more because of various environmental factors and people's lifestyle. The similarity of both systems today is what we now define as internal medicine. Both the Chinese Medicine

Chapter Three: Comparison of Traditional Chinese Medicine and Western Medicine

and Western Medicine had a basis and model when it comes to understanding human nature. At the dawn of the 18th century, Chinese Medicine was regarded as more advanced than Western Medicine because it is more organized and systematically developed.

This chapter will show you the significant difference as well as the many similarities that both of this ancient medical systems share so that you can better understand how they can complement one another.

Western Medicine vs. Traditional Chinese Medicine

One of the fundamental incompatibilities between Traditional Chinese Medicine and Western Medicine is that the former has only limited pathological and also anatomical knowledge. Chinese Medicine's theory is different than Western Medicine, fundamentally speaking.

The rise of Western Medicine around the 19th century has outdated some principles of Traditional Chinese

Chapter Three: Comparison of Traditional Chinese Medicine and Western Medicine

Medicine. For instance, the development of microscope gave scientists detailed information of the organ and cell's microscopic structures. This led to the introduction of the cell as the center of the body's changes pathologically. This outdated the TCM's view that illnesses are due to the imbalance of the 4 humors. From then on Western Medicine linked the patient's diseases to cellular pathological process and also linked such changes to the physiology and also chemistry of the body. Western Medicine made huge and significant advances when anesthesia and surgery became recognized in 1846 through various methodological research and also scientific work. And because of this, Chinese Medicine became somewhat stagnant because it cannot show scientific proofs of its abstract ideas. Western Medicine up to this day is the most exact medical system ever developed even if has its shares of flaws. Scientists and doctors of Western Medicine have used these flaws to developed a much better approached that gave birth to other fields of science like biochemical, biological, genetics, and other branches of sciences we now have today.

Chapter Three: Comparison of Traditional Chinese Medicine and Western Medicine

Western Medicine is more population based and it uses theories of reductionism while Chinese Medicine tends to be more holistic in its approach. This holistic approach in Traditional Chinese Medicine follows Aristotle's concept in Metaphysics which is "the whole is more than the sum of its parts," wherein the medical system views the different part of the body as a whole organ, and it also emphasizes the coordination of each internal parts as well as other body structure, and at the same time unites the body with the external environment. Thus, Chinese medicine is more concerned in the unity of the body, mind, and spirit. The idea behind this is that the person is in a constant battle of opposing forces (based on their yin and yang theory) such as hot and cold, happiness and sadness, and the likes. And if there's an imbalance in such factors it can ultimately cause a person to become ill or susceptible to external conditions. Therefore, the goal of Chinese Medicine is to restore the body's imbalance. It aims to focus not just on the causes of the symptoms but also how the whole body system is affected by such illnesses unlike in Western Medicine where it only focuses on the symptoms of the particular organ or

Chapter Three: Comparison of Traditional Chinese Medicine and Western Medicine

body part that is affected, and only applies individual organ treatments. There is no singular factor in Chinese Medicine compared to the philosophies of Western Medicine.

In Chinese Medicine, if an individual is sick, the whole body must be treated so that the person can fully recover. There's also no such thing as single diagnosis unlike what Western Medicine does. You won't get the same kind of treatment in Chinese Medicine because this system believes that the patient's condition is constantly changing, which is why treatment is based according to the development of the condition. This is what makes Traditional Chinese Medicine both a homeostasis and a homedynamics medical system.

One of the similar things between the two systems is how it identifies the classification of the disease. Just like in Western Medicine, Chinese Medicine uses listening, smelling, inspection of body parts, and the pulse palpation to gather information about the possible illness. The main difference though is that in Western Medicine, once a patient is diagnosed, it is often a result of one pathogenic factor. An

Chapter Three: Comparison of Traditional Chinese Medicine and Western Medicine

example of this is if a patient has lung problems, Western Medicine will tell you that the possible cause is harmful microorganisms, the diagnosis will not likely change even after the commencement of antibiotic treatments. Compared to Traditional Chinese Medicine, a disease can be caused by both a pathogenic factor AND the maladjustment of the patient which means that the condition will constantly change during the illness' course. According to Chinese Medicine doctors the number of potential stimulants is huge but the body's reactions are limited. In Chinese Medicine, visible signs and symptoms are usually analyzed in order to identify a pattern of syndrome. This pattern of syndrome means that the functional state is the combination of both the body's response and also the pathogenic factor, this is why the treatment given in Chinese Medicine is designed to improve a person's regulatory mechanisms, and also aims to remove various factors that can hinder the self – healing abilities of the body.

Although different illnesses have various pathological factors, the response of a body varies in different people, and

Chapter Three: Comparison of Traditional Chinese Medicine and Western Medicine

therefore requires a different therapy or treatment. However, Chinese Medicine doctors still give individualized treatment/ therapy based on the patient's constitution and its symptoms.

The Chinese Medicine's pattern of syndrome is not explained in a conventional way (anatomical/ physiological) but instead it's explained through a philosophical thinking path (yin and yang; 5 elements theory; and qi). This is where Western Medicine collides with Chinese Medicine. Western Medicine explains the connection of pathology and anatomical/ physiological changes, on the other hand, Chinese Medicine relies on empirical knowledge and also philosophical thinking. TCM focuses more on the function than the structure which also came from Taoism and culture origin in ancient China.

The challenge of Traditional Chinese Medicine today is to prove its efficiency because it is quite difficult to evaluate and also research due to its different principles and abstract theories.

Chapter Three: Comparison of Traditional Chinese Medicine and Western Medicine

Chapter Four: Basic Theories of TCM: The Yin - Yang Theory

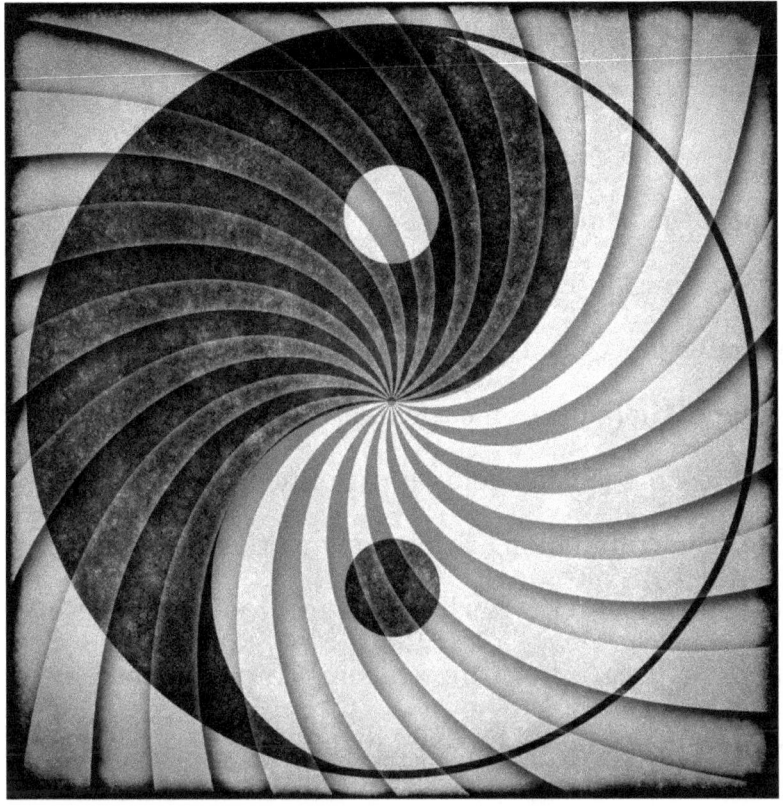

Traditional Chinese Medicine in its form came from the philosophies of ancient China, and is further influenced and developed by the accumulated medical experiences of various practitioners. And although Chinese Medicine is sometimes outdated because of its cultural context, it is still a complete and integrated method when it comes to

Chapter Four: The Yin – Yang Theory

understanding the physiological and pathological changes in an individual's body.

The most important ideology taken from the ancient Chinese philosophy in Chinese Medicine is Qi, Yin – Yang, and also the 5 Phases. Other theoretical concepts used in Chinese Medicine are the Zheng Ti Guang Nian doctrine, Zangfu Xue Shuo (viscera and bowels), Jingluo (channels and network), Qi Xue Jing (body fluids, substances, blood), and Bing Yin (pathogenic agents). These theories combined with the 4 diagnostic methods of Si Zhen as well as the pattern discrimination are the framework that Chinese Medicine is based on. Each therapeutic tools of Chinese Medicine like acupuncture, Zhenjiu, Chinese herbology/massage is also based on these theories.

This chapter and the next will cover two of the most important theories where Traditional Chinese Medicine is anchored on. The first one is the famous Yin – Yang Theory or YingYang Xue Shuo.

Chapter Four: The Yin – Yang Theory

The Yin – Yang Theory

This theory represents the universal standard of quality that is both complementary and opposite in nature. The Ying – Yang is used to describe a function, and the relationship of each as part of the constant change and transformation in the universe. When applied to medicine, it is used to compare and also contrast as well as differentiate a physical and pathological condition.

Yin is often associated with qualities like responsiveness, passive, cold, dark, interior, downward, inward, decrease or other similar meanings. Yang, on the other hand, is associated with the opposite which is movement, heat, light, exterior, activity, stimulation, upward, increase and outward motion. It's very important to note that such aspects only happen in relation to one another. For example, the absence of heat is known as cold, the absence of light is darkness etc.

In medicine, this theory is usually applies as opposites; Yin is the body's structure, and Yang is the body's function. The lower body part is Yin, and the upper part is

Chapter Four: The Yin – Yang Theory

Yang. Such concepts though are never absolute. It is only applied in objects to express its relationship to one another.

The 4 Fundamental Characteristics of Yin – Yang Theory

- Opposition
- Interdependence/ Relativity, and Interdivisibility
- Inter – Consuming – Supporting
- Intertransforming

Opposition

As mentioned earlier, the Yin – Yang theory is mostly described as an opposition. The Yin aspect exists because of the Yang aspect and vice – versa. It presents a certain duality of the universe. Common examples are heaven and earth, male and female, inside and outside, night and day etc. Another classic example to illustrate this characteristic is water and fire. Water is cold, fire is hot. Water flows downward while fire rises. In the Yin – Yang theory, Yin is water and fire is Yang.

Chapter Four: The Yin – Yang Theory

In medicine, the anterior side of the body is Yin, and the posterior is Yang; the medial aspect of the body's extremities is Yin, and the lateral aspect is Yang. The body's interior is Yin, and the exterior is Yang. The zang/ viscera organ which are considered solid is Yin while the fu/ bowel organ is Yang. Diseases that manifest hot or excessive symptoms / activity are Yang; on the other hand, illnesses that manifest cold symptoms are Yin. Rapid and forceful pulses are Yang while slow and forceless motions are Yin.

The table below is the basic Yin - Yang correspondence that is being used in Chinese Medicine.

Yin	Yang
Water	Fire
Qi	Blood
Cold	Hot
Right side	Left side
Interior	Exterior
Medial aspect of the limbs	Lateral aspect of the limbs
Slow	Fast
Anterior region	Posterior region

Chapter Four: The Yin – Yang Theory

Passive	Active
Dimness	Brightness
Lower body	Upper body
Stagnant	Movement
Inhibition	Excitement
Structure	Function
Internal organs	Body extremities
Hypoactivity	Hyperactivity
Structure	Function
Interior	Exterior
Downward motion	Upward motion
Zang organs	Fu organs

Interdependence

Yin and Yang depend on each other and it also represents the aspects of the whole. The "whole" is something that's defined as the existence of 2 opposing aspects. They mutually define one another.

In terms of medicine, Yin – Yang interdependence is the structure and function's relationship. The structure is

Chapter Four: The Yin – Yang Theory

Yin, and the function is Yang. They complement one another and are essential to the whole – which is the human body. The body fluids, cells, tissues, etc. allows the body to function normally, but it is only when the functional processes are in good condition can such substances be rightly replenished. The balance achieved in the body's structure and function is the main basis of a healthy physical body.

Interdivisibility and Relativity

Yin – Yang cannot be solely labeled as something purely Yin or Yang. No even or phenomenon can do it because it highly depends on the viewpoint of the analysis. For instance, day is Yang, and night is Yin but the early hours in a day is Yang, and the hours after noon are Yin. In Chinese philosophy, morning is referred to as Yang within Yang, and afternoon is Yin within Yang. And such hierarchies can be extended infinitely and also divided in both its Yin and Yang aspects.

Inter – consuming – supporting

In Yin – Yang theory – gain, advancement or growth of one aspect also means the loss, retreat or decline of another. This is known as the waxing and waning of the Yin and Yang. In physiological terms, it is like homeostasis. There are certain limits, and if it exceeds, the results could be a dysfunction or a disease in the body.

For instance, a Yang illness, say an excess in metabolic activity will slowly consume the Yin (or resources) of an individuals' body. Advanced age (Yin) can bring forth a reduction in one's body function (Yang). In pathology, all illnesses are thought of as the body imbalances, and excess of Yang/ excess of Yin; deficiency of Yang/ deficiency of Yin.

Intertransformation

The Yin and Yang implies a constant transformation which can be observed. Yin transforms into a Yang, while Yang evolves into a Yin. The Yang day becomes a Yin night, similar to the shadows moving in the face of a hill as the sun travels across the world.

Chapter Four: The Yin – Yang Theory

In medicine, intertransformation of this Yin and Yang happens in 2 ways; development and death. There's the growth and aging, and then there's death and internal imbalance in response to the changes in the environment.

Usually, Yin and Yang follow one another, and is always in a state of constant transformation. The success process is pertained to as health, while disease is what happens when this very process is disrupted when the Yin and Yang are out of balance.

According to Chinese medicine, when Yin reaches the extreme, it will naturally transform into Yang. Similar to when heat blazes, it transforms into something cold.

Yin –Yang Theory Application to Chinese Medicine

As what the previous examples have shown, the Yin – Yang theory is used as a framework in understanding the various branches of physiology, pathology, anatomy as well as diagnosis and treatment.

Chapter Four: The Yin – Yang Theory

Chapter Five: Basic Theories of TCM: The Five Phase Theory

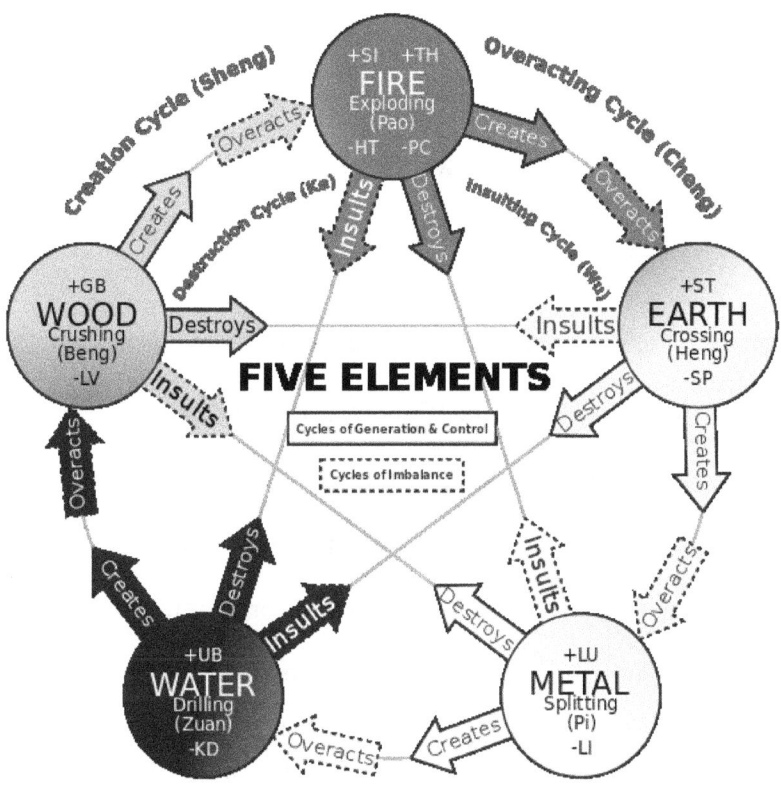

Another very important theoretical framework in Traditional Chinese Medicine is the 5 Phases or the Theory of Five Elements. This is a very complex system of body correspondences that shouldn't be viewed in absolute. As you can see in the photo above, the 5 – star configurations

Chapter Five: The Five Phase Theory

are visualized and represented by 5 elements: Fire, Metal, Earth, Wood, and Water. Each of these elements also corresponds to the Yin and Yang organs. The Yin pertains to solid organs while the Yang pertains to hollow organs. This chapter will give you an overview of the 5 Phase theory and its application in Chinese Medicine.

The 5 Phase Theory and Its Body Correspondences

For instance, the Earth element includes the spleen which is also a Ying organ, while the Yang organ is the stomach. Each of these organs has its own functions in Chinese Medicine that greatly varies from their physiological functions in the Western system counterpart. There are 12 organs that are associated with different tissues, emotions, color, sound, direction, season, spirit and other correlations. See the table below as the reference for each elements and body correspondences.

Chapter Five: The Five Phase Theory

	Wood	Fire	Earth	Metal	Water
Direction	East	South	Center	West	North
Climate	Wind	Heat	Dampness	Dryness	Cold
Season	Spring	Summer	Late Summer	Fall	Winter
Number	8	7	5	9	6
Planet	Jupiter	Mars	Saturn	Venus	Mercury
Cereal	Wheat	Millet	Sorghum	Rice	Beans
Meat	Chicken	Goat	Beef	Horse	Pork
Sound	Jiao	Zheng	Gong	Shange	Yu
Color	Green	Red	Yellow	White	Black
Musical Note	C	D	E	G	A
Taste	Bitter	Acid	Sweet	Pungent	Salt
Smell	Uremic	Burnt	Scented	Cool	Putrid
Organ	Liver	Heart	Spleen	Lung	Kidney
Viscera	Urinary Bladder	Small Intestine	Stomach	Large Intestine	Bladder
Sense	Eyes	Tongue	Mouth	Nose	Ear

Chapter Five: The Five Phase Theory

Organs					
Bodily Sounds	Hu (sigh)	Laugh	Singing	Crying	Moan
Tissue	Tendons	Vessels	Muscles	Skin	Bones
Virtues	Benevolence	Courtesy	Fidelity	Justice	Knowledge
Emotion	Anger	Joy	Worry	Melancholy	Fear
Bodily Region	Neck or nape	Thorax	Spine	Escapulodorsal	Lumbar
Spiritual Activity	Hun	Shen	Yi	Po	Zhi

Endangering Cycle

This is the cycle whereby the process is believed to proceed for it to generate one another in a sequence that is of order. This goes to show that the natural movement of 1 phase fosters the growth or waxing of the next. For instance, the wood engenders the fire while the fire engenders the earth, the earth engenders the metal elements, the metal engenders water, and the water engenders the wood. This is also known as the Mother – Son cycle or relationship. The engendering phase is acting as "mother" to the next which is the "son."

This cycle is very relevant in diagnosing and also treating patients. For instance, a cough may not be caused by a metal pathology but could be from the Earth element, which means that the treatment that should be given to the patient aiming to not just treat the metal but also nourishing Earth.

Controlling Cycle

This cycle follows the sequence of which the phases are controlled or suppress each other. As an example, the wood controls the earth, the earth controls water, water controls fire, the fire controls the metal element, and metal controls wood.

Chapter Five: The Five Phase Theory

For instance, treating a heat disorder/ disease (like insomnia); you can supplement water to ease this heat problem and/or modulate a person's restlessness.

This means that through the 5 phase system, the organs of the body are intertwined thus disease in one body part can affect another. This also means that all phases stand in relationship to one another in 4 ways: engendering, being engendered, controlling, and also being controlled. It means that the state in 1 phase is always dependent of the other phases' conditions. If it is viewed as part of an organic whole, then the actions of engenderment and also control that is being exerted in each phases can add up just to maintain a balance.

Application in Chinese Medicine

The 5 phase correspondences can be applied to Traditional Chinese Medicine. The Zang (Viscera) and the Fu (bowels) along with the pressure points is classified in this system of the 5 phase correspondences. The 5 phase theory is also used to understand the physiological and pathological system of the human body in relation to its external environment. It can also be applied in diagnosis, prognosis and treatment.

The main 5 phase correspondences that are used in Chinese medicine is those of the Zang organs; wood is the liver which regulates the Qi flow in the body; fire element is attributed to the heart that provides a warming source of the body; the earth is the spleen which is responsible for the transportation of the food digested and also its transformation into the energy that the body needs; the metal is attributed to one's lung which promotes the Qi's descend; the water is the kidney or the renal organ that is in charge of storing and regulating body fluids.

Below is the basic engendering and controlling relationships of the 5 phases in the physiological aspect:

Chapter Five: The Five Phase Theory

Engendering Cycle

- **Wood engenders fire:** The liver stores blood and it also supplements the blood that is regulated by the heart.
- **The Fire element engenders the earth:** The heart (fire) promotes warmth in the body that is used by the spleen to function properly.

- **The earth engenders the metal element:** The spleen transports and transforms the needed nutrients and sends it up in order to replenish one's lung.

- **The metal engenders water:** The lung using its clearing function sends the fluids down to the renal organ.

- **Water engenders wood:** The kidney nourishes the blood in the liver.

Chapter Five: The Five Phase Theory

Controlling Cycle

- **Wood controls the earth:** The liver's effect prevents the spleen from becoming stagnant.

- **Fire controls metal:** the heart's upward and outward movement prevents the lung from descending excessively.

- **Earth controls water:** The spleen's transportation prevents the fluid in the kidney from overflowing.

- **Metal controls wood:** The lung's action counteracts the liver's ascent

- **Water controls fire:** The kidney flows in an upward movement that nourishes the heart thus restricting it.

Chapter Five: The Five Phase Theory

The Use of 5 Phase Theory in Diagnosing Symptoms

The correspondences of the 5 phase theory are very useful when analyzing symptoms. Chinese medicine needs to correlate data in order to arrive at a certain diagnosis which means that within this context, the actual meaning of one symptom may differ when analyzed in relation to the whole problem. There are other signs such as facial complexion, tone of voice, body odor etc. which can be used as indicators of illnesses that affects the corresponding attribution of the 5 phase theory or the associated organ, which is why sometimes it can be used to construct a medical strategy using the engendering and controlling cycles in therapy.

Five Phases Applied in Therapeutics

There are certain pathological conditions that are the result of an imbalance between 2 or more body organs. This is based on the clinical researches done by doctors wherein they find that symptoms and signs occur together which are

Chapter Five: The Five Phase Theory

also associated with certain conditions of the Chinese medicine diagnostic theory.

That being said, treatments should focus on regulating such relationships. In some cases, it means that the affected organ or phase should be treated. A very effective therapeutic strategy is the "Mother and Son" relationship. Similar to an old adage, if there's an excess, tonify the Mother, and drain the Son.

When applied in clinical practices, one should tonify the kidney to help heal the liver's deficiency. However, majority of the 5 phase based therapeutic strategies used in the modern Chinese medicine involves using a special group of pressure points known as the *shu* points.

Chapter Five: The Five Phase Theory

Chapter Six: Chinese Medicine and Chronic Diseases

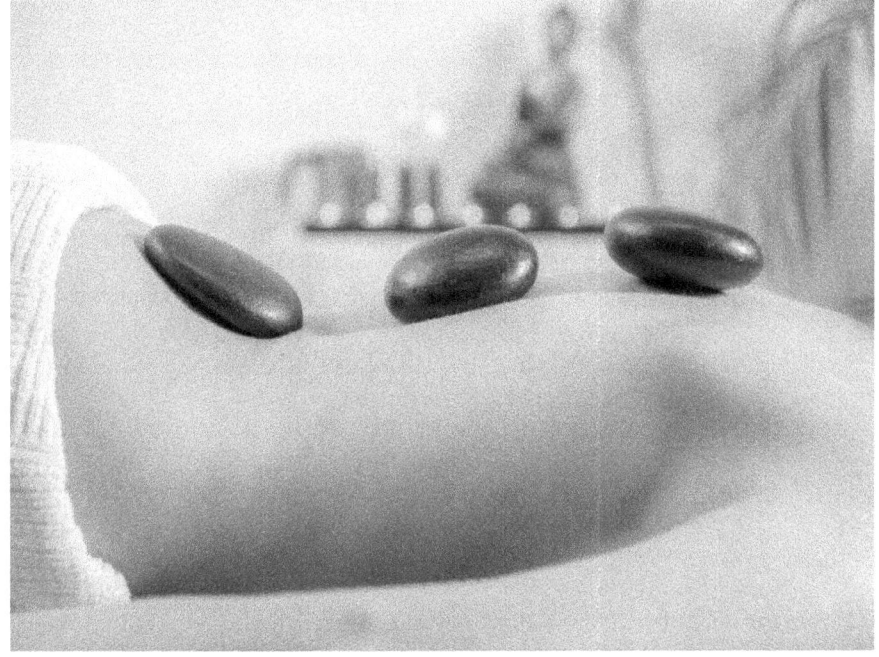

There are many Chinese medicine practitioners and also patients who claimed that the treatment methods of this medical system are very helpful against fighting chronic or recurring diseases. The Chinese have the opportunity to choose both the Western Medicine and TCM whenever they are stricken with an illness and most of them through years of experience and disease encounters have concluded that Chinese medicine and Western Medicine is better and much

Chapter Six: Chinese Medicine and Chronic Diseases

more effective when combined as it helps heal a person physically and holistically.

TCM and Chronic Diseases

Most patients believe that Chinese medicine is a good use for both minor illnesses and chronic diseases such as colds, coughs, and other musculoskeletal disease. TCM is best known for getting to the root of an illness when the surface level or physical methodologies of Western Medicine fails. Chinese medicine is also a great supplement to get rid of some side effects caused by Western Medicine medications.

When it comes to implementing treatment such as medications, most Chinese people will agree that TCM is much slower and takes a long time to prepare such as in the case of herbal medicines. It's also bitter and usually unpleasant when applied. Some TCM practitioners will also ask their patients to avoid eating certain types of food during the course of the treatment as some foods can

Chapter Six: Chinese Medicine and Chronic Diseases

aggravate the disease. As mentioned earlier, it's part of Traditional Chinese Medicine philosophy that the treatment given to the patients should depend on the present condition or progress of the disease because an illness to them is constantly changing. This makes the practice of Chinese medicine a bit difficult because the patients will need to go back and forth (which is time – consuming for most people) when seeking the treatment until the disease is healed.

Most patients particularly in Asia both seek Western and Chinese medicine during the course of their diseases. Usually, if they are stricken with mild illnesses like a cough, patients will try to use herbal medicine first but if the illness didn't get any better then they'll consider seeking Western medicine types of treatment as it is much faster than using herbal medicine though not always as effective. The usual purpose is for the patient to gain control of the symptoms until they get well, once the Western medicine does that, they usually go back to TCM in order to tackle the root cause of the cough or the disease.

Chapter Six: Chinese Medicine and Chronic Diseases

As people age, chronic disease is something that's causing a great burden to many people and also health care systems. Doctors of Western Medicine and their patient often aim to get effective and fast treatment. When it comes to TCM, there had been many systemic researches done to show the efficacy of this system and how it can cure chronic diseases through herbal medicines and other therapeutic methods like the popular acupuncture as it has shown many benefits like reducing lower back pains, eliminating tension – type headaches, chronic neck pain, arthritis, osteoarthritis, migraine, heart diseases, eczema, and type 2 diabetes to name a few.

In Europe like in Germany, there are now many hospitals have provided TCM based therapies aside from Western medicine. And even if there are no exact proofs or scientific evidence supporting the TCM's efficacy, many foreign patients are still considering trying Chinese medicine. And most of them after the treatment were convinced that Traditional Chinese Medicine is just as beneficial as the Western Medicine therapies especially for

Chapter Six: Chinese Medicine and Chronic Diseases

patients suffering from neurological and musculoskeletal illnesses. Chinese medicine therapies is said to have improve the quality of life among patients but more research is still required to address the effects of Traditional Chinese Medicine especially in relation to various chronic diseases.

TCM and Organ Diseases

The concept of organ diseases in TCM is very different from the Western medicine's understanding wherein organs have energetic functions that may or may not be entirely related to the body's physical functions. For instance, if a person has a kidney disease, A TCM doctor wouldn't imply that the patient needs dialysis, he/she only diagnoses that the energetic qualities of one's renal organ is weak which is why it's affecting the main function of the kidney (to regulate water metabolism, stores essential nutrients, governs head hair, bones, marrow etc. filters body fluids). Another example is if a child is experiencing chronic fear which in TCM is associated with the Water element, the child might complain of having or experiencing enuresis,

Chapter Six: Chinese Medicine and Chronic Diseases

he/she will attempt to cure it with words but wouldn't be effective if the root cause is deficient kidneys.

In this context, TCM points out that all organs in the body have certain functions and also energetic abnormalities that can have an adverse effect to other organs of the body. All organs are also associated with respective elements, and also the 5 phases as well as the Yin – Yang theory.

There are many etiological factors and patterns that can be found in organ diseases; in the context of traditional Chinese medicine, it can be caused by the following:

- 6 External Pathogenic Influences and the 7 Emotions
- 6 External Causes (Heat, Wind, Cold, Summerheat, Dryness, Dampness)

Each of these influences can attack and weaken the human body especially if the immune system is not strong. Such influences can also translate into different pathogenic – related attacks in the form of viruses, bacteria, fungi and other microorganism.

Chapter Six: Chinese Medicine and Chronic Diseases

Emotional Instability

One major factor that can lower the immune system of a person according to TCM principles is emotional instability. In Chinese medicine, the 7 Emotions are the following:

- Joy
- Grief
- Fear
- Fright
- Sadness
- Anger
- Worry

If there are any excess or even absences of such emotions, it can be damaging to the respective organ. Translating such emotions can cause organ disharmony; for instance, sad experiences can cause lung infections because the sadness emotion decrease the respiratory systems defense mechanism thereby making a person susceptible to air – borne illnesses. In ancient Chinese, this phenomenon is

Chapter Six: Chinese Medicine and Chronic Diseases

known as the "evil Wind" has invaded a person's body making the lung's capability to weaken; hence the person is coughing or will experience suffering colds.

Other usual causes of illnesses is a result of consuming too much alcohol, eating too much "cold" or "hot" foods or over – indulgence of the five flavors which is also links to the 5 Elements that can injure the respective organs associated with it. For instance, too much sweets intake will cause stomach or spleen damage; too much salt will affect the kidneys and could lead to edema.

Much like in Western Medicine, TCM has its own set of medical specialties. These are the following:

Nei Ke (Internal Medicine)

- Gynecology
- Pediatrics
- Ear/ Nose/ Throat (ENT)
- Opthalmology
- Urology

Chapter Six: Chinese Medicine and Chronic Diseases

- o Psychiatry
- o Neurology
- o Geriartrics
- o Oncology

Wai Ke (External Medicine)

- o Orthopedics
- o Trauma Medicine
- o Dermatology

Diagnosis of Organ Diseases

In TCM, diagnosis is done through the use of the 4 Inspections; these are inquiring, visual inspection, listening and smelling, and palpation to gain information and gauge the patient's problem. It also involves asking the patient where it hurts, knowing about the medical history, psychological factors, and other related issues as these can all be part of the explanation as to what might be the root cause of a particular illness or disease. If you go to a TCM

Chapter Six: Chinese Medicine and Chronic Diseases

doctor, don't be surprised that he/she will pretty much follow the same methods of diagnosing used in Western Medicine like inspecting your tongue, nails, hair, checking your heart rate, breathing, and pulse etc. as these can all provide a clue (especially the tongue and pulse) regarding a patient's pathological issue or state. A normal tongue for example is pink in color and has a normal size as well as a thin white coat, if there's a pathological issue, the color could be reddish, pale or purple with either a narrow size, a swollen appearance, or too wet/ dry. It can also show a sticky or slimy surface.

It's the same with the pulse rate, TCM doctors will measure both the radial artery found in the wrists or in the carotid. The normal pulse rate according to TCM is 60 to 80 beats per minute. The rapid changing of the pulse can also be used as verification system. After the treatment, the patient's pulse rate should achieve a balance or be one with the normal harmony of the organ system. Such patterns of disharmony will be discussed in the next chapter.

Chapter Seven: Patterns of Disharmony

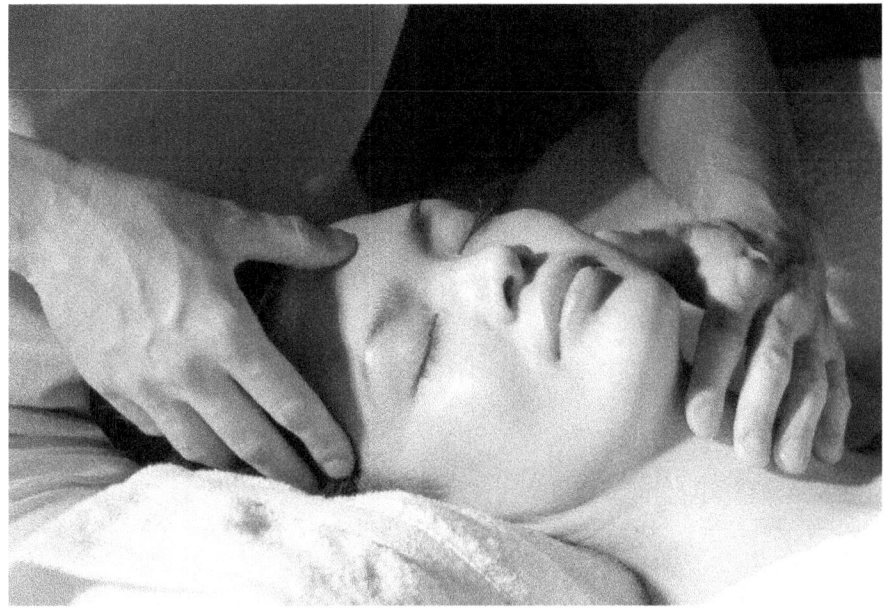

When a patient has been examined by the Chinese Medicine doctor, he/she will give a diagnosis, say for example, asthma, and also the so - called pattern of disharmony (ex: Lung deficiency resulting to colds or cough may have underlying Kidney deficiency). If the Yin and Yang are in perfect equilibrium, the Qi and the blood flows smoothly and efficiently throughout the body because there's sufficient amounts generated, as a whole the individual is considered healthy.

Chapter Seven: Patterns of Disharmony

This chapter will discuss an overview of what the pattern of disharmony is all about and its significance in Traditional Chinese Medicine.

The 8 Yin and Yang Pathologies Diagram

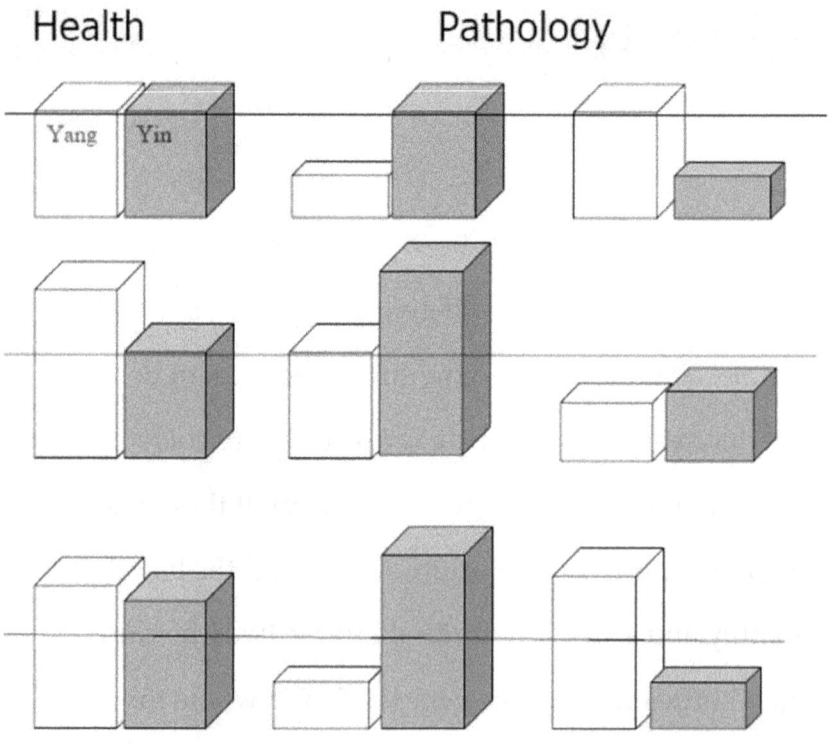

Chapter Seven: Patterns of Disharmony

Whenever Yang is deficient, the person would appear having more Yin qualities; an individual may feel that he/she is experiencing colds, feeling lethargic, has a frail pulse or pale – colored tongue, or even a lowered sex drive. But if Yin (cooling agent) is deficient, there might probably be an excess of Yang; an individual may tend to be more sexually driven, might become restless at night, may feel signs of dryness, and has thin pulse rate and perhaps a reddish tongue.

In such a case where Yang is excessive than the Yin, the individual or patient may have gotten an invasion from the external Wind Heat which is why he/she might be experiencing a high fever. If for example, a person with an excess in Yin got wet in the rain, and he/she wasn't able to immediately change his/her wet clothes then he/she may suffer acute edema.

Another example is if a person has osteoporosis; most TCM doctors will view this as deficiency in the person's Yin and Yang; Yin (which associated with the bone) is diminishing, while Yang (function of the bone) is also losing its primary function which is to carry the body. In such a case, if both the Yin and Yang is excessive, then the patient may experience some form of damp heat, according to TCM philosophies related to the elements. It may be manifested as acne, and in the case of dampness and heat it can exhibit signs of pus, bad odor, redness or discharge.

Finally, if the Yang is deficient and the Yin is excessive, then the patient might exhibit obesity, coldness, or phlegm nodulation which is usually seen in persons with Polycystic Ovarian Syndrome (PCOS). On the other hand, if the patient has hypertension, menstruation that is ahead of schedule (with other symptoms like burning sensation, red face or blood – shot eyes), or experiencing headaches that usually means, according to TCM, an excessive Yang, and a deficient Yin.

According to Chinese Medicine, all these diseases or disorders manifests as an imbalance energy or what they call a pre – morbid condition before it manifests into a pathologically morbid condition which can be confirmed

Chapter Seven: Patterns of Disharmony

and measured later using the Western medicine's diagnostic methods.

Such imbalances in the energy can be distinguished as the Chinese medicine's way of examination or diagnosis. There are 3 phases of the pre – morbid and morbid conditions totaling into 6 phases:

Pre – Morbid Conditions	Morbid Conditions
Phase 1: There are no OM patterns of disharmony which means that the patient is healthy and its energy is in perfect balance	**Phase 4:** There are now obvious OM patterns of disharmony; the person is ill, and there are mild/ abnormal results in Western medicine's diagnostic methods through findings in blood work or imaging; medications are given.
Phase 2: The person is healthy but experiences mild	**Phase 5:** The patient is exhibiting severe OM

Chapter Seven: Patterns of Disharmony

symptoms from time to time; there might be a visible but mild OM patterns of disharmony which won't be recognized yet by the objective methods used in Western Medicine.	pathological patterns of disharmony; there's now abnormal diagnostic results found through lab work. Aside from medication, surgery may be needed from the view of Western medicine physicians.
Phase 3: There are visible patterns of disharmony in OM but may still not being recognized by Western Medicine; patients are now experiencing visible signs or serious complaints.	**Phase 6:** Patient is very sick and can be terminally ill; may need to be in the Intensive Care Unit (ICU).

Such patterns of disharmony as well as their respective treatment plans will guide a TCM practitioner in resolving the patient's issues and also help in dealing with their own diseases during the entire course of it. In TCM,

Chapter Seven: Patterns of Disharmony

there are various treatment modalities that a patient can choose such as the following:

- Acupuncture
- Acupressure
- Chinese Herbal Therapy
- Moxibustion (Artemisia burning or leaf preparation)
- Cupping (suction of cups that's applied to the body to draw out pathogenic influences), Tui Na (massage), diet therapy, Qi Gong/ Tai Qi (breathing exercises/ gentle movements)

Example of Patterns of Disharmony

To further elaborate the patterns of disharmony, the example that will be given in this section is those patients experiencing or about to experience menopausal. The Yin, Yang, Qi, and Blood is what Chinese medicine physicians use to diagnose different menopausal manifestations, similar to how they diagnose other diseases as what you've read earlier. The chart below will show you the Yang excess, Yin

Chapter Seven: Patterns of Disharmony

deficiency, Qi stagnation, and blood deficiency as well as the Yang deficiency, Yin excess, Qi deficiency, and Blood stasis. The Yin, Yang, Qi, and Blood may all exhibit in different diseases which mean that there's a need for diagnosis and treatment to be according to the patient's condition.

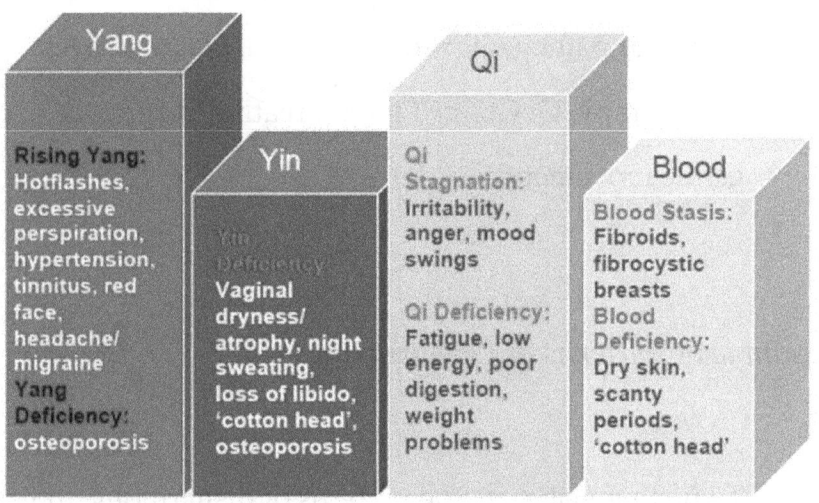

Chapter Eight: Acupuncture

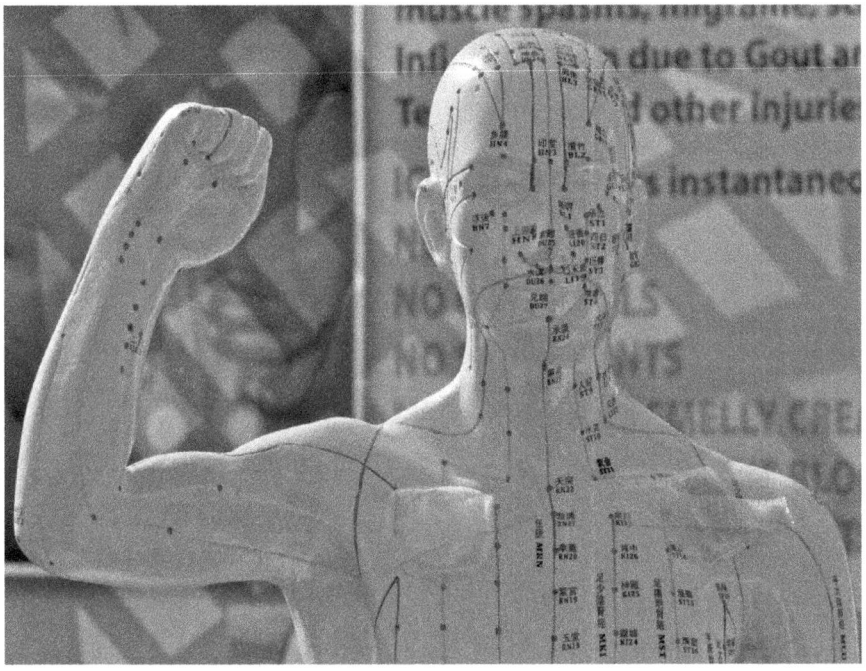

Acupuncture is another main pillar of the Traditional Chinese Medicine philosophy. It is derived from the Latin word "acus" which means needle, and "pungere" meaning to punctate. In Chinese terms, it is known as Zhen Jiu; Zhen (needle), and Jiu (warming – a technique used when applying acupuncture). Acupuncture has been one of the subjects being studied in Western Medicine for a long period of time now. As a matter of fact, it is now an accepted form of therapy in many countries because it has many benefits

Chapter Eight: Acupuncture

and also a good complementary and alternative method of therapy.

This chapter will provide you with the basics of acupuncture and how it is crucial in the field of Traditional Chinese Medicine.

Brief History of Acupuncture's Development

In Chinese medicine, there are also the so – called 12 main meridians which are correlated to the 6 Yin and Yang organs, and there's also the 8 Extra Meridians. The Qi flows from one of the organ meridian to another in a certain order until all of the networks or the meridians in the body are covered delivering vital energy forces to each body parts. Chinese medicine doctors use the Qi flow with acupressure/acupuncture along with the meridian network in order to influence the whole body.

There's an ancient old reference written around 762 A.D. called Ling Shu (Vital Axis), and in this book, there are around 365 pressure points that are being utilized. However,

Chapter Eight: Acupuncture

we now know that there are over 2,000 pressure points in the body. Acupuncture and also moxibustion reached the west during the 17th century through the Japanese.

Moxibustion is the ancient process involving Chinese herbal medicine. It is the burning of dried Artemisia leaves on the skin surface of the person. These leaves were rolled into a cone and are usually pressed on the acupuncture point so that it will provide a warming sensation in a particular region of the body. The term moxibustion came from the Japanese word called "Mogusa" which means burning of herbs. The process of Moxibustion is also used back then to turn a fetus in a pregnant woman who has been detected with breech presentations.

Each pressure points in acupuncture has different functions. There are points that regulate one's digestion, promote labor, calm the spirit, relieve body pain, and improve blood circulation as well as supplements the Qi, Yin, Yang, and the Blood etc. Needles in the past were made out of flint and thorns from various plants like bone or

Chapter Eight: Acupuncture

bamboo silvers. Today, modern TCM practitioners use pre – sterilized stainless steel needles.

In the West, Acupuncture reached in the U.S. when President Richard Nixon went to a trip in China around the 60's and witnessed how acupuncture anesthesia was successfully used during a surgical operation when one of his colleagues needed to get his appendix removed. The president also saw how it helped in the post – surgery when managing pain. Since then, acupuncture was introduced to the west, and was utilize by many patients. Today, there are around 300,000 physicians in 140 countries that use acupuncture as part of the treatment plan. 15,000 of this came from the U.S., and now there have been various styles of acupuncture developed throughout the world. These are the following:

- Traditional Chinese Medicine
- 5 Element Acupuncture
- Japanese Acupuncture
- French – Style Acupuncture
- Vietnamese - Style Acupuncture

Chapter Eight: Acupuncture

- Korean - Style Acupuncture

Each of style has its own way of using acupuncture in diagnosing and also treating a patient. You can see the various medical acupuncture styles on the next page.

Traditional Chinese Medicine

Methods of Diagnosis: 4 Methods of Examination (Patterns of Disharmony)

Use of Herbs: Yes

Needling Method: Tonification, sedation, strong stimulation, deeper insertion with gauge (28 to 34 needles). Needles are usually retained for up to 45 mins. Point selection depends on the point actions and indications.

5 Elements or Classical Acupuncture

Methods of Diagnosis: 4 Methods with primary focus on pulse (all disease has emotional etiology)

Chapter Eight: Acupuncture

Use of Herbs: No

Needling Method: Mostly tonification technique; Insertion of needles is 1 to 2 mm deep (using very thin needles). Feedback system is via pulse diagnosis. Point selection according to Constitution al Factors, point names, and 5 element points. Needles retention time varies from 5 sec to 15 minutes.

Japanese Style Acupuncture (Matsumoto)

Methods of Diagnosis: Palpation of various religions, zones, pulse and tongue

Use of Herbs: Yes (using Kampo system)

Needling Method: Mostly tonification technique; Insertion of needles is 1 to 2 mm deep (using very thin needles). Feedback system is via pulse diagnosis or abdomen. Also uses of intradermals, magnets, and ion pumping cords.

Korean Style Acupuncture

Methods of Diagnosis: Patient involves dividing them into 8 constitutional types. Acu – formula for each type.

Use of Herbs: Yes

Needling Method: Horary points serves as transmitter; 5 elements points as receiver.

Vietnamese Style Acupuncture

Methods of Diagnosis: Excess of deficiency within 5 element diagram; it's made according to symbol of a tree.

Use of Herbs: Yes

Needling Method: Tonification and sedation techniques

Classical Balance Method

Methods of Diagnosis: Primarily based on Yi Jing; 4 methods of examination

Use of Herbs: Yes

Chapter Eight: Acupuncture

Needling Method: Tonification and sedation techniques. Point selection according to 6 Division channel associate.

French – Style Acupuncture

Methods of Diagnosis: Based on 6 Divisions and Yi Jing

Use of Herbs: No

Needling Method: Tonification and sedation techniques Point selection accdg. to Ying Jing trigrams, 5 Elements and 6 Six Divisions common use of electro – acupuncture for analgesia.

Significant Researches on Acupuncture

One of the very first studies that were done in order to capture the scientific basic of acupuncture was published sometime in the 70's. A group of researchers used a model of severe pain that was caused by potassium iontophoresis with also gradual increase of electrical current. Volunteers of the experiment will be given acupuncture in the large intestine and stomach, as well as IM morphine. It is done in

Chapter Eight: Acupuncture

a random way. The results showed that the acupuncture and the administration of the morphine increased the volunteers' pain threshold by an average rate of 80 to 90%. However, when the investigators injected the local anesthesia in the subject's acupuncture points, it became quite ineffective in increasing the subject's pain threshold. The result of the experiment suggested that in order for the transmission of acupuncture signals to be evident, the sensory nervous system must be intact.

Intensive experiments and research is continuously being done to demystify the acupuncture's working mechanism. As what most researchers have found out, the most significant effect of acupuncture is its analgesic function which is mediated by the different neurotransmitters in the body's central nervous system. There are also studies that proves acupuncture have some local effects, as it has already been a great treatment for someone experiencing lower back pains. The main treatment consists of pressure points as well as the so – called Ah Shi

Point. This Ah Shi Point is a functional point near the site where the pain is being felt.

According to recent studies, an acupuncture needle can stimulate the nerve fibers in the muscles and can also trigger the release of vasoactive substances that can improve the blood flow and promotes healing. Other studies also show that the needle activates nerve fibers in the spinal cord.

Acupuncture treatment is now ranging from various disorders such as the following:

- Lower back pain
- Chronic Asthma
- Rheumatoid Arthritis
- Vascular Dementia
- Epilepsy
- Migraine Prophylaxis
- Nausea/ Vomiting caused by chemotherapy
- Insomnia
- Smoking cessation
- Psychological disorders like schizophrenia and depression

Chapter Eight: Acupuncture

How to Receive Acupuncture

Acupuncture needles are usually fine, thick, and flexible with average lengths of around ¼ inches to 1/5 inches long. In general, needles are inserted just below the skin's surface, though the needles may be inserted in deeper areas of the body. Acupuncture won't resemble of the feeling of being injected since injections' main pain point is its hollow needle and the medication is usually forced into the tissue through pressure. In acupuncture, the needles are used to disperse energy along the body's meridians, and not merely for injecting. Various needle techniques are usually applied to these pressure points that are based from traditional Chinese medicine and the TCM practitioners' diagnosis and treatment plan.

Many patients find the acupuncture therapy very relaxing and not painful at all (since it's a form of therapy) and it brings a feeling of great well – being. Some people experience a slight feeling of sensation when a needle is

Chapter Eight: Acupuncture

being inserted in the skin but when the needle reaches the Qi or the pressure point.

Some patients report that they feel a hot or cold sensation along the body's meridian pathway from the needle that is placed on that meridian point.

Statistical studies have shown that acupuncture reveals that it is very safe because the needles placed don't cause any form of severe bleeding or extreme bruising. Many TCM practitioners will make appropriate referrals to Western doctors to further diagnose a disease or do some form of lab work if it is deemed necessary. There are many patients see their western doctors simultaneously TCM physicians.

The question now is how the manner of sticking needles stimulates the body's energy and moves it along certain pathways and specific nerve channels? How does it move from the organs to the skin surface and the tissues?

According to research, the mechanisms of the Qi are still something that needs to be demystified. In the western

Chapter Eight: Acupuncture

medicine point of view, it is still theoretical, though there had been some progress when it comes to sorting out the hypothetical factors of acupuncture's therapeutic effects.

Acupuncture has clinical value for different kinds of illnesses. In the United States, it is popularly used for treating musculoskeletal conditions, joint pains, nerve pains and other neurological disorders, compared to China where it is used as a modality for diagnosing a patient's disease using different treatment methods such as the respiratory, urinary, digestive, gynecology, and emotional disorders etc.

Acupuncture has shown positive results for the following disorders:

- Nausea
- Diarrhea
- Allergies
- Cough
- Vomiting
- Constipation
- Frequent urination
- Urinary incontinence

- Anxiety
- Painful menstruation
- Depression

Most mild complaints may provide immediate relief when acupuncture is applied but chronic and severe illnesses may tend to take some time to improve. Usually, chronic illnesses take years before the patient restores a certain balance. Acupressure can also be used on the patient if the person is sensitive to needle. Most of the time pressure points are massaged, and acupressure has milder effects compared to acupuncture.

For ear acupuncture, TCM practitioners use small needles and insert it in the different ear points that can be left for quite some time. Recently, ear acupuncture is used to treat patients suffering from addiction as it can be used to adjunct to the different pressure points in the body.

Chapter Nine: Traditional Chinese Medicine and Cancer

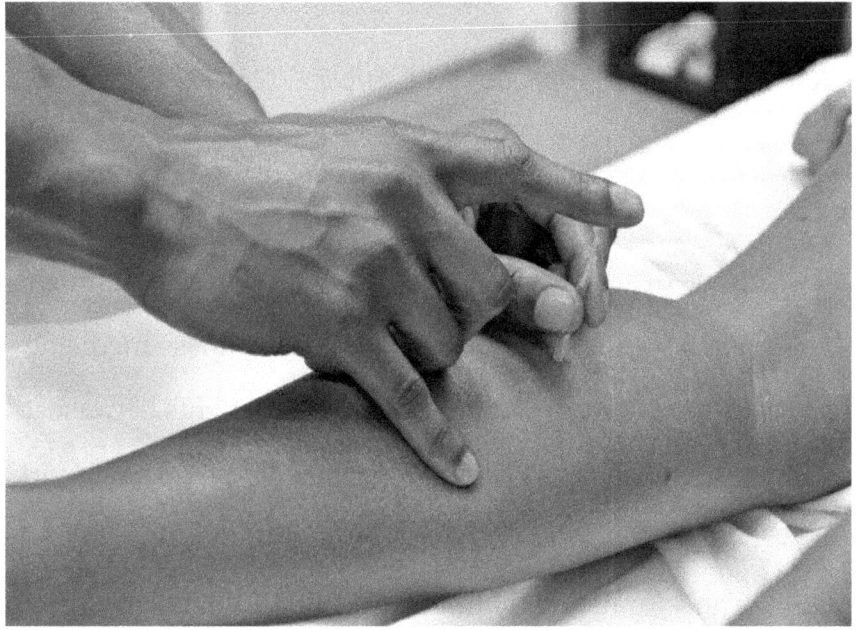

Cancer is one of the most common illnesses of this century. It's also one of the most stressful experiences a patient can have. Once diagnosed, patients and physician's alike come up with a coping strategy to not just ease the pain but also change the current lifestyle of the patient – perhaps to a much healthier one. This is why most cancer patients are advised that even after they have recovered from the illness, they should maintain a healthy lifestyle by having a strict

Chapter Nine: Traditional Chinese Medicine and Cancer

balanced diet, exercise, intake of vitamins and other nutritional supplements, doing meditations and the likes.

TCM's Holistic Approach to Cancer

According to the principles of Chinese medicine, viewing the deadly disease holistically can enhance a much better health for the patient which is why Chinese medicine is becoming more popular among cancer patients because it is the next best alternative if Western medicine doesn't work.

Cancer patients who seek traditional Chinese medicine thinks that the system can detoxify one's body, make the symptoms more manageable, boost one's immune system, boost the energy, reduce the possible side – effects or adverse effects of the anti – cancer treatments given in Western medicine, and also maintain a good quality of life. There are also lots of people who believe that TCM can slow the cancer's growth and perhaps prolong one's life since most patients are aware of the disease's incurable nature.

Chapter Nine: Traditional Chinese Medicine and Cancer

In Chinese medicine, the treatment to cancer and also its complications is mainly consisting of application of Chinese herbal medicine, diet, and acupuncture. The medical system is obviously focusing on the body and mind network. In TCM, the malignant tumor that is also common when diagnosed with cancer is considered as the stagnation of both the Qi and the Blood. As you now know, Qi is viewed as an ancient model for intracellular and also intercellular information transfer. If a patient has cancer, Qi is stagnated because the intra and intercellular information in the body is disrupted. The key therefore is de – stagnation to treat it.

One of the most common terms in TCM treatment is Fu Zheng (Correcting to the normal). This treatment aims to strengthen the body and mind system through enhancing and also harmonizing the energetic balance in all the organs. This is also often viewed by TCM physicians as correcting the body and mind communication network and its imbalance which is also reflected through enhancing one's

Chapter Nine: Traditional Chinese Medicine and Cancer

immune system. Fu Zheng includes Chinese herbal medicine like the following:

- Astragali membranaceus
- Paeoniae rubrae
- Ligustici Chuan xiong
- Angelicae sinensis

The molecular basis of such medicines has been suggested as the induction of cancer cell apoptosis, anti-angiogenesis promoting immunologic response to cancer cells, regulating oncogene expressions. Aside from herbal medicines, TCM doctors also focuses on the cancer's other aspects including its various physical illnesses such as exhaustion, pain, fatigue, nausea, psychological problems etc. which can be caused by either the disease itself or the side – effect of the treatment given, or sometimes both.

Using acupuncture therapy could also be an effective treatment to patients experiencing mild depression, and it can also be effective in managing short – term pain. Different

Chapter Nine: Traditional Chinese Medicine and Cancer

cancer types also use different kinds of Chinese herbal medicine and it's also effective in treating vegetative symptoms.

As more and more patients take traditional Chinese medicine in combination with western medicine, patients also need to be aware of the possible side-effects of it. Some side – effects of TCM may include abnormal liver function tests, unexpected severe myelosuppresion, haemostatic defects, or renal functional impairment.

Many Chinese medicine physicians claim that by using the right herb patients, patients would gain benefits such as myeloprotection, hepatoprotection, neuroprotection, nephroprotection, and also gut mucosal protection. What went wrong was that Western Medicine practitioners have to apply to herbs according to Chinese medicine diagnosed criteria.

According TCM doctor Tai Lahans, she describes one of her patient's encounters with integrating Chinese medicine and Western medicine treatment. The patient is diagnosed as colorectal cancer with Duke's stage C adenocarcinoma;

Chapter Nine: Traditional Chinese Medicine and Cancer

Lahans also gives the patient a diagnosis based on TCM principles which is "above plus damp heat with Liver and Kidney Yin deficiency." The patient was treated with Western Medicine surgery, and undergone chemotherapy for about 3 weeks after the surgery. What is special is that the patient received TCM deduction pre and post - surgery. The treatment all in all was successful and the patient is now cancer free 10 years later. This example tells us that whether we view the disease from the Chinese medicine perspective or conventional point as in the case of Western medicine treatment, the patient is still the same. Both TCM and Western medicine are the health care system we make in our attempt to understand the human body.

Chapter Ten: Chinese Herbal Medicine

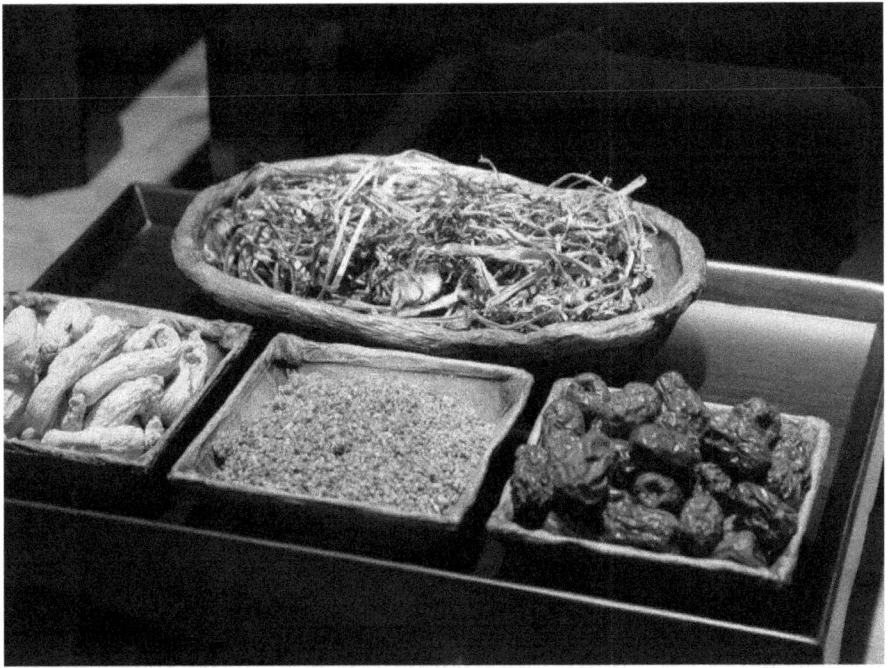

Within the context of Traditional Chinese Medicine, the Chinese Herbal treatment/ therapy is perhaps one of the oldest methods of treatment in the world, and today it is becoming more and more popular especially as an aid in Western Medicine. This chapter will provide you with a wealth of information that you need to know regarding Chinese herbal medicine, including its brief history of how it came about and how it was developed, its different classifications, its comparison with synthetic drugs usually

Chapter Ten: Chinese Herbal Medicine

prescribed in the West, and the different ways on how to administer it to the patient.

Brief History of Chinese Herbal Medicine

Shen Nong (3737 – 3697 B.C.E) is one of China's legendary emperor about 5,000 years ago. He is said to have become fascinated with the medical uses of different herbal plants and how it can help heal various types of diseases or mild injuries. His research and work is all included in the classic Chinese herbal medicine book called *The Shen Nong Ben Cao Jing – Classic Materia Medica*, which was later published around 200 B.C. E. According to historians, the emperor has personally tried for himself the different medical properties that each plant has to offer. As a matter of fact, he listed 360 herbal medicines in his book and also its uses – both the good and bad. Yes, that includes poisonous plants! Most of the herbs he tried are part of the Plant Kingdom, but there are also some that came from animals and minerals.

Chapter Ten: Chinese Herbal Medicine

A thousand years later, many ancient Chinese medical practitioners have discovered many more functions of these herbal plants, discovered more than what the emperor originally tried for himself, and they also have passed it on from one generation to the next. With the advent of books and written works, various Chinese scholars have documented everything that they have researched about regarding the good and bad benefits of herbal medicines to certain types of illnesses, and have also discovered how much one should use or apply depending on the patient's condition. One of the most notable books is published during the Warren States era (475 to 221 B.C.E.) called *Nei Jing*. A few years later, a famous TCM doctor by the name of Zhang Zhong Jing, who witnessed first – hand the death of people caused by various infectious diseases, had written another book entitled Shan Han Lun (Treatise on Febrile Diseases Caused by Cold).

Around 200 A.D. Hua Tuo was the first one to use narcotics, through his so – called "narcotic soups" to his patients in order to manage or relieve pain. And because of its success, around 1200 A.D., practitioners have started giving "narcotic teas" to their patients after undergoing minor surgical procedures.

During the Song Dynasty (960 – 1279 A.D.) the pharmacopoeia that encompasses around 1,000 substances was taken from either different plants, minerals, animals, or a combination of the three; Pharmacopoeia is the compilation of all the standardized herbal plants prescriptions, research regarding the collecting and preparing of different herbal medicines, research about toxicity, and the instruction and guidelines on how to prepare and apply herbal pills, pastes, and poultices on different kinds of ailments. From this day forth, the idea of using herbal plants as medicines spread from China to other parts of Asia.

In 1590 A.D., another Chinese scholar and TCM practitioner, by the name of Li Shi Zhen compiled the most important research regarding herbal medicines in his book called Ben Cao Gang Mu (Grand Materia Medica). There are about 52 volumes of this book, and is now known as the

Chapter Ten: Chinese Herbal Medicine

cornerstone Chinese herbal medicine. The book covers around 1,800 substances and over 10,000 traditional Chinese medicine herbal formulas. The book was later published in other parts of the world.

When Prostestant missionaries introduced the use of Chinese herbal medicine to the West in 1700, the usage of these ancient medicines declined but when China established their new government called the People's Republic of China in 1949, Chinese medicine and herbal medicines became popular again, and was also integrated into mainstream health care, since then the art and science of using Chinese herbs to cure various ailments and diseases spread throughout the world and is now being used to complement Western medicine.

In 1977, Jiangsu College of New Medicine published a book called Zhong Yao Da Ci Dian (Encyclopedia of Traditional Chinese Medicine Substances). The book covers aroun 5,700 single substances that is both the culmination of efforts of scholars dating back many millennia and the new generation of TCM practitioners. Each herbal medicine in the

Chapter Ten: Chinese Herbal Medicine

book is thoroughly described and other parameters were also included like the descriptions regarding the plant's taste, indications, and actions as well as the different dosage recommendations, preparations and also the possible contraindications.

Today, the Chinese people managed to fully integrate both the traditional Chinese medicine and Western medicine. There are about 40% of Chinese who uses herbal medicines as their primary health care modality. Many TCM practitioners are trained in both Chinese medicine and Western medicine, which is why patients are usually cross – referred to both medical systems as they view both health care systems as complementary.

Classification of Chinese Herbs

Similar to the different function of acupuncture points wherein it is use to correct the Qi's flow through the body, Chinese herbs or herbal plants also functions as such within the context of Chinese pharmacopoeia. As you may now know in traditional Chinese medicine, different organs,

Chapter Ten: Chinese Herbal Medicine

tissues and sense organs are all attributed and link to the 5 Elements which is why each Chinese medicines are classified into different taste and also temperatures within this context. The 5 tastes into which Chinese herbs are groups are the following:

- Pungent
- Sour
- Bitter
- Salty
- Sweet

Similar to eating chili peppers, a person can be caused to break out into a sweet herb because it can either cool or warm the person down. Chinese herbs can be hot, warm, slightly warm, neutral, slightly cool, cool, or cold. Warm medicine will treat cold conditions, and cold medicines can also treat heated patterns or illnesses; making the herbs both warm in temperature and pungent in its taste. Chinese medicines are classified into different types (to name a few):

- Herbs that can harmonize one's digestion
- Herbs that stop cough
- Herbs that promote urination
- Herbs that resolve phlegm
- Herbs that quicken the blood's circulation
- Qi Supplement

Emperor Herbs: Major herbs containing bioactive components for any pathophysiological diseases or conditions.

Minister Herbs: Herbs that provides support for the Emperor herbs' action. It alleviates secondary symptoms of illnesses.

Assistant Herbs: This serves as the modulator of the actions of major herbs. It also enhances the action, and counteracts possible side – effects of herbal mixture.

Messenger Herbs: These herbs direct the action of other kinds of herbs aforementioned to the specific body parts and organs.

Chapter Ten: Chinese Herbal Medicine

Compared to Western medicine, the Chinese herbal medicine approach focuses more on the importance of the ingredient's balance and interaction than the effect of a single ingredient; it focuses more on the whole. Western medicine will usually prescribe 1 or 2 herbal ingredients, in traditional Chinese medicine; the prescription will usually contain 40 herbs or more that each has unique and different chemical compositions. Traditional Chinese medicine is actually based on the principle that every medicinal ingredient has its own strengths and also weaknesses, which is why it should be carefully balanced in terms of the quantity and quality of the ingredients used. It should also be formulated in a way that it would increase its efficacy, and at the same time have little to no side – effects to the patient. The main difference of a good TCM doctor versus an amateur practitioner is their ability in synergistically makes each herb ingredients cooperate with one another in terms of their beneficial usage without jeopardizing the patient. The most essential factor in achieving success in TCM is to treat each patient as an individual.

Chapter Ten: Chinese Herbal Medicine

Herbal medicines include ingredients that come from all the parts of the plant including the flowers, leaves, and roots. It can also include ingredients from animal substances like rhinoceros horns, seahorses, tiger bones and the likes.

Chinese Herbs vs. Synthetic Drugs

It's essential that you understand the difference between a Chinese herbal medicine (ex: ingesting the mineral, animal or plant substance), and the western pharmacological approach (reduction of a substance to its active ingredient). In Western medicine, a plant substance is usually taken, and what pharmacists/ scientists do is find the active ingredient in the plant that can be used in treating certain illnesses. After doing that, they'll extract that active ingredient/s and make it concentrated or refined.

In China, if a medicine is effective in treating not just one illness but a lot, then it is considered superior. The more disease it treats, the more useful it is and beneficial to people. One of these very useful herbs is known as the Radix Ginseng. It is a tonic to many body systems, and a very

Chapter Ten: Chinese Herbal Medicine

precious medicine in China. However, the medical term 'tonic' doesn't exist in Western medicine concepts and philosophies which is why this herbal medicine may not be considered as something superior, that's the same in Chinese medicine, a synthetic drug may not also be considered superior and vice – versa. As what you now know, traditional Chinese medicine follows the natural way, and has a much broader approach to treating diseases. It also prefers the gradual way, and looks at treating diseases as treating the whole body.

Another great example of Chinese herbal medicine is ephredine. It came from the Chinese herb called Ma Huang or Herba Ephedrae. In Western medicine, this herb was refined and concentrated into a synthetic drug, and use as a treatment for patients with asthma. However, the side – effects of this if it was turn into a synthetic form is that it can overstimulate a person's heart, increases heart rate and nervousness, and it can also contribute to high blood pressure. In TCM, this herb is used in its raw form, and ephedrine's concentration is only 1%. The beneficial effects

Chapter Ten: Chinese Herbal Medicine

of this herb when it is in its raw form are gradually metabolized since the plant has buffers that sort of eliminate its possible adverse effects. Nevertheless, the use of this plant can have many great benefits but should also be used with caution. Long – term usage or overdosing it is not recommended. According to the book of Chinese Materia Medica, the intended use for this herbal plant is to dispel the Wind Cold to treat the colds of asthmatic patients, therefore it shouldn't be used in 'herbal uppers' or as pills to say, reduce weight.

The process of only concentrating the active ingredient of a medicinal herb has become very popular in the Western medicine. However, the moment that such active ingredients are isolated, then it's no longer considered an herb but rather a drug, at least according to Chinese medicine philosophy. Generally speaking, medicinal herbs works in a more gentle and gradual way but may not be recommended for very severe conditions or something that needs immediate solution. Most of the patients seeking

Chapter Ten: Chinese Herbal Medicine

herbal medicines are those with recurring illnesses or chronic diseases.

Preparation of Chinese Herbal Medicine

There are many ways to prepare a Chinese herbal medicine. The most common way of preparing is as follows:

- **Infusion:** This is quite similar to just making a cup of tea. You just have to boil the water, and pour the different herbs, and just kept it covered for at least the next 10 to 15 minutes.

- **Decoction:** Very similar to the process of infusion, but the only difference is that the herbs is boiled for a much longer period of time.

- **Tincture:** This is when water and alcohol is extracted in order to make the plant soluble in water. Some plants have very active chemicals that make it hard to

Chapter Ten: Chinese Herbal Medicine

boil them. This method is also used when preparing for a bigger quantity or if it needs to be stored for a long time. There are many properly tinctured plants that can last for many years without losing its potency. It is a very common belief in China that the more tinctured the plant/s gets the more potent and beneficial. The longer it is stored the better it becomes.

- **Maceration:** It is the process of covering the plants and soaking it in cool water overnight. After which the herb should be taken out and strained so that the liquid can be used. This is usually the method done for plants that are fresh or those with naturally delicate chemicals that might be gone or degraded if it was heated or mixed in with strong alcohol.

Traditional Chinese medicine nowadays has already taken another form like pills, capsules, tablets, and plaster that are used to relieve pain. There are many herbs and dried ingredients that are now turn into pills. They usually

Chapter Ten: Chinese Herbal Medicine

look like round black pills like an M&M shape chocolate. Some of these medicines are mistakenly called patent medicines but in reality it's not really patented in a sense that there's no standardized formula in it. All Chinese "patent" medicines usually have the same amounts of ingredients but no one has exclusive right to the formula as what real patented medicines bear. Chinese patent medicines such as those herbal medicines in the formed of pills or capsules are much easier to take and convenient. However, these are not easy to individualize in patients which is the fundamental principles of traditional Chinese medicine. Such preparations though are best applied if the condition of the patient is not severe, and the preparation is also best use if it is taken as a treatment for the long run.

The main challenge perhaps of Chinese herbal medicine is its consistency. TCM herbs are quite complex because there are different kinds of plant species, cultivation herbs, time of harvest which can lead to variations in its raw quality. Herbs can have more than one active ingredient which further complicates its variation in terms of bioactive

Chapter Ten: Chinese Herbal Medicine

components and composition. Varied concentration of such bioactive components can either lead to the under dose or overdose to a patient.

The herb's chemical composition can also be altered by its method of preparation. The good thing is that despite of its complex nature, Chinese herbal medicines have attracted many western pharmaceutical companies. They use it to discover natural bioactive components. Bioactive compounds became a critical issue when it comes to developing new herbal products. There had been many scientific ways to identify different herbs. Some methods include electrophoretic methods, spectroscopic methods, and chromatographic methods.

Fingerprinting method is also becoming quite popular recently; however it doesn't promote the usage of techniques though it encompasses a different style of data evaluation. Fingerprinting technique is the combined methods of chromatographic, electrophoretic and spectroscopic method. It also establishes a herbal pattern that's based on its similarity and also integrity.

Chapter Ten: Chinese Herbal Medicine

Types of Herbal Administration

There are many TCM practitioners that use pre – packaged herbal medicines in the forms of pills because patient compliance is much better since it's more convenient to carry around and easy to administer. The main challenge however is the individual customization of such prescriptions to patients, and the efficacy of the plant may tend to be weaker than herbal decoctions. Herbal medicine is usually administered to infants and elderly as freeze – dried plants. Granules are also quite advantageous because it's much easier to administer and also comes in the form of capsules. The processing of creating these herbal medicines and turning it into synthetic forms can greatly increase the price, thus the debate arising whether or not capsule forms are equally effective than decoctions methods.

Chinese medicines are usually used for different kinds of diseases and ailments. A few examples of conditions/ illnesses where herbs are often used are sore throat, fatigue, dysmenorrhea, allergies, frequent urination,

Chapter Ten: Chinese Herbal Medicine

incontinence, bowel syndromes, edema as well as anxiety and depression.

Once the pattern of disharmony and also a treatment plan was established by the TCM doctors, a herbal medicine formula is carefully customized for the patient. It's important to note that no 2 patients will have the same amount and schedule of prescription as it will depend on their conditions at the time. For instance, if there are 5 patients who have the same diagnosis, they'll most likely get different kinds of herbal medicines and formulas that are tailored according to their varying patterns of disharmony. This goes to say that Chinese herbal medicines shouldn't be prescribed without first seeing a professional TCM doctor as the patient will need to be thoroughly checked first, and must be in accordance with the patient's condition at the moment. Herbal medications usually involves a combination of different plant varieties like dried twigs, seeds, flowers, roots, fruits, barks and other animal/ mineral components.

There are around 90% Chinese medicines that are plant based. Of course, the best herbs are naturally grown in

Chapter Ten: Chinese Herbal Medicine

China, and the increasing demand in herbal medicines, and the increasing popularity of traditional Chinese medicine has now become a booming agricultural industry in the country. The parts of the plant that are being used from various medicinal purposes differ according to the herbs. Some plants only use the roots while others use the stem or the fruits, still others use almost all parts like the leaves, flowers, seeds etc. as each have its own medicinal value. After being harvested, they are usually dried. Different substances that go with it should also be carefully prepared (ex: herbs that are cooked in vinegar, cut in a certain way, boiled or even fried with honey). These are sometimes done so that the plants can achieve its highest medicinal state.

Animal substance are less commonly used because people wanted to protect such species, substitutions are usually done as much as possible. Animal substances are traditionally used and are even considered to have strong medicinal qualities. They are usually found in patent types of medicines (herbal medicines in the form of pills, capsules

Chapter Ten: Chinese Herbal Medicine

etc.) but it only uses a small amount in order to conserve such animal species.

Chinese medicine doctors who are based in the West usually use herbal medicines as a treatment modality. Usually after doing decocting methods, the herbs are then given to the patient in the form of a tea as a main method of administration so that the patient can quickly absorb the ingredients and create an immediate effect. When a patient takes herbal medicines for a particular disease, he/she can be treated with it daily, and may just require fewer acupuncture treatments which can be cost effective in the part of the patient. All in all, herbal medicines enhance the TCM treatment, and also aids in the patient's speedy recovery.

Important Basic Concepts to Remember in Traditional Chinese Medicine

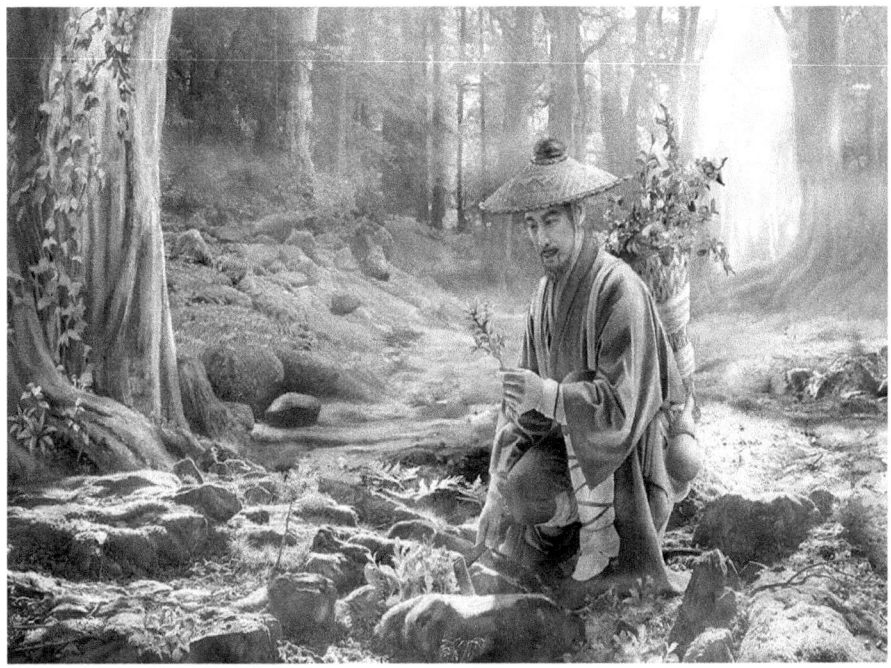

It takes experience to get good at practicing the art and science of Traditional Chinese Medicine. The important things are that it may have initiated a thought process in you in a way that you start thinking about things not in terms of diseases. As you now have learned, Western medicine tends to think things in terms of diseases, and just throw a remedy at this particular illness; in Chinese medicine what they do is treat the individual or the person and not the illness that the person has. It's very intriguing because Chinese medicine practitioners are always treating not the disease but the underlying energetic imbalance in the body which is causing that particular disease, which could be in one person's case; say an excess/ lack thereof of Yang or a deficient/ excessive Yin. If you understand that the solution lies in looking not just at the particular present symptom but the overall pattern of symptoms of the body – not just the physical ones.

Important Concepts

- In this world, everything has a force. If there's a force in one hand, there's a counter – balance force on the other hand, and those two forces kept in balance is what sustains life and what sustains creation.

- The symptoms of deficient Yang includes cold limbs, cold aversion, tendency for swollen tongue, tendency of impotency or lack of sexual desire as well as loose stool or undigested food.

- Blood deficiency is very important because in Chinese medicine, you have Chi and Yang associations, and Blood and Yin associations. Chi is the life energy, blood is the physical energy. If blood is deficient you have a tendency to have thin and emaciated body, have tremors in limbs, have a dry skin or lackluster complexion, impaired vision, and also thin pulse. The remedies that usually build the blood is herbal medicines like beet root, burdock, I – X and Chinese Build Blood formula.

- The symptoms of deficient Yin are pretty much the same as blood deficiency with warm sensations in the palms and also the feet, insomnia, thirst and also agitation. Yang deficiency is an exaggerated chi deficiency, and Yin deficiency is an exaggerated blood deficiency.

- The common Chinese medicine remedies that build Yang includes Korean ginseng, ginger, kidney activator, trigger immune, capsicum, garlic and parsley. On the other hand, the remedies that build Yin include Licorice, Marshmallow, American ginseng etc.

- The symptoms of excess and deficient are another important principle in TCM because it can be used as a guide in selecting the right remedy.

- The common symptoms of Excess are generally acute, it includes a person with heavy discharge through sweat, diarrhea, mucus discharge, vomiting etc., excess dampness or heat and also stagnation or body congestion. On the other hand, when a person is in the deficient state the symptoms are generally

chronic, weak, lethargic, light discharge, lacks energy such as fluids, low grade chronic inflammation, and also loss of muscle tone.
- In order to balance excess, you have to clear or reduce the excess which is equivalent to the western medicine concept of cleansing – getting rid of the excess or discharging the excess heat, mucus or toxins. In deficient conditions, you have to nourish and strengthen the body in order to overcome the deficiency or in the west, it's known building.

- Reducing formulas to reduce the excess includes anti – gas formula, liver balance, stress relief, kidney activator, mood elevator etc., building formulas to aid the body's deficiency includes spleen chi activator, blood build, nervous fatigue formula, trigger immune.

- Heat is a manifestation of Yang, and cold is a manifestation of Yin. A person can't get excessively hot or excessively cold. Symptoms of heat include inflammation, redness, fever, irritability, aversion to heat, rapid pulse, red tongue, burning sensations. Symptoms of cold include slow pulse, paleness, poor digestion, aversion to cold, heavy white coating on the tongue etc.

- The remedies that reduce heat includes Aloe Vera, Thai – go formula, VS – C formula, IF – C formula. The remedy that's needed to warm up cold conditions includes ginger, trigger immune, capsicum and spleen activator.

- Pernicious Environmental Influences (also known as "evils")
    - Wind: movement and tension
    - Heat: moves up and out, hyperactivity
    - Cold: congeals and contracts
    - Dampness: heavy. Wet
    - Dryness: lack of moisture

Wood Element (Symbols of Energy)

- This is associated with the liver organ and also the gallbladder. The liver is the Yin wood element, and the gallbladder is the Yan wood element.

- The emotion associated with the wood element is anger. An excess of anger damages the liver and gallbladder.

- The Wind evil tends to damage the wood element

- The wood element nourishes the blood and connective tissue; if the blood and connective tissue is deficient, then it is a deficiency in the wood element

- The taste of the wood element is sour

- Symptoms of excess wood include vomiting, diarrhea, constipation, nausea, headache, fatigue in the morning, bitter taste in the mouth, achy muscles, grogginess, anger/defensiveness. Symptoms of deficient wood include hypoglycemia, moodiness, depression, skin infections, frequent fatigue, difficulty in waking up or getting to sleep, discouraged feelings, hypochondriac feelings.

- Remedies that reduce wood element include dandelion, red clover, liver balance, and Oregon grape; remedies that increase wood are Chinese Blood Build formula and green veggies.

Fire Element (Symbols of Energy)

- Fire as an energy affects the heart (yin) and small intestines (yang) as well as the nervous system of the body.

- The emotion associated is joy and excitement

- The evil that damages the element is heat

- It also builds arteries in the body, and the taste is bitter.

- Symptoms of excess fire include excitable, anxiety, dizzy, nervous, restlessness, too much stress, people who talks too fast, highly emotional symptoms. Symptoms of deficient fire include cold hands/ feet, loss of sexual drive, confusion, restless dreams, forgetfulness, feeling burned out, night sweats.

- Remedies that reduce fire element include hawthorn, chamomile, nutria – calm, Stress – J formula. Remedies that increase fire include Schizandra berries, Nervous Fatigue formula, and adrenal support.

Earth Element (Symbols of Energy)

- Earth elements are associated with stomach (yang) and spleen (yin) organs.

- The emotion that damage the earth element are worry and sympathy

- The "evil" that damages the earth are humidity and dampness

- It also builds muscles, and the taste is sweet.

- Symptoms of excess earth include bad breath, sugar cravings, belching after every meal, bloating, foul taste, temporary loss of appetite, sour tummy, acid indigestion. Symptoms of deficient earth include low energy levels, shallow breathing, poor protein digestion, intestinal irritation, poor or thin muscle tone/ unable to gain weight, loos of energy, poor appetite

- Remedies that reduce earth element ginger, Chinese Anti – Gas formula with Lobelia, Catnip and fennel. Remedies that increase earth include juniper, spleen Chi activator, saw palmetto, American ginseng, proactazyne plus.

Metal Element (Symbols of Energy)

- The organs associated with the metal element are the lungs and colon.

- The emotion that damages the metal element are sadness and grief

- The "evil" that damage the metal element is dryness.

- It builds the skin and hair; it is pungent in taste.

- Symptoms of excess metals include acute respiratory, asthma, coughing, sinus headaches, swollen lymph glands, difficulty breathing, allergies, hayfever, sneezing, sinus congestion, and excess of mucus production. Symptoms of deficient metals include chronic lung infection, chest tightness, tuberculosis, tends to be withdrawn making a person "cold," wheezing, lung weakness, dry cough, emphysema, lack of power or feeble speaking.

- Remedies that reduce metal element garlic, onions, and ginger, AL – J formula. Remedies that increase metal include Cordyceps, American ginseng, and astragalus.

Water Element (Symbols of Energy)

- The organs associated with the water element are kidneys and bladder

- The emotion that damages the water element is fear

- The "evil" that damage the water element is coldness

- It builds the bones, and the taste that nourishes the water is salty.

- Symptoms of excess water include edema, sluggish, prostate swelling, frequent urinations, burning urine and UTI, pale urine, backache, fearfulness, timid, and joint swelling. Symptoms of deficient water include neck pain, gout, arthritis, impotency, osteoporosis, weak ankles, legs, and knees, spinal misalignment, dark circles under the eyes, stiff neck.

- Remedies that reduce water element include Juniper, JP – X, Kidney Activator, and Chinese Kidney Activator formulas. Remedies that increase water include horsetail, goldenrod, nettles, KB – C formula.

Conclusion

In TCM, doctors also look at an individual's emotional state as this is a great guide in selecting the appropriate remedies because if for example, you're looking to treat someone who's angry all the time, then you need to give medications that may reduce that energy or element to balance out the body. Understanding these methods will help you see the interplay between a human's physical and emotional nature. The underlying connection between the physical and emotional is energy. Energy underlies the emotions as well as the physical processes and functions of the body. Seeing this different opposing forces of the body (hot/cold, damp/dry, excess/deficient etc.), and seeing where this thing is in excess or that thing is lacking will determine what you as a potential TCM practitioner will nourish or reduce certain processes to bring the energy level of the body back into balance.

At first, TCM principles may seem confusing especially if you're someone who grew up learning the conventional way of the health care system which is Western medicine. It might take you a while to grasp it but as you work with it and learn more about it, you'll realize that it's much easier for you to study the different methods than learning about hundreds of different diseases and try to figure out therapeutic protocols for them because you're not looking at the disease, you're looking at a person who has the disease, and try to find ways of balancing their energy so that their physical body and emotional state is also energetically brought back in harmony or balance.

TCM is about looking at the bigger picture. It's all about learning to think in a different way, and like most things in life, all it takes is some practice and experience. We hope that as you go through this book and ponder the concepts and principles given here find that the ancient secrets of traditional Chinese medicine are very valuable in helping you understand better the modern health problems through learning the important lessons of being balanced, and also learning to work on the person not on the disease.

Photo Credits

Page 10 Photo by user bomb_bao via Flickr.com,

https://www.flickr.com/photos/bomb_bao/4596065926/

Page 17 Photo by user jo3f via Flickr.com,

https://www.flickr.com/photos/jo3f/2744516004/

Page 21 Photo by user clairegren via Flickr.com,

https://www.flickr.com/photos/clairegren/2381320772/

Page 27 Photo by user Nicolas Raymond via Flickr.com,

https://www.flickr.com/photos/80497449@N04/8691983876/

Page 35 Photo by user Manonastreet via Wikimedia Commons,

https://commons.wikimedia.org/wiki/File:FiveElementsCycleBalanceImbalance_02_plain.svg

Page 48 Photo by user white session via Pixabay.com,

https://pixabay.com/en/massage-massage-stones-welness-2717431/

Page 54 by user Kai Miano via Pixabay.com,

https://pixabay.com/en/massage-wellness-japanese-1929064/

Page 72 Photo by user Denver Aquino via Flickr.com,

https://www.flickr.com/photos/denveraquino/4385199696/in/photolist

Page 81 Photo by user Massage Nerds via Pixabay.com,

https://pixabay.com/en/acupuncture-asian-medicine-needles-2277444/

Page 91 Photo by user mac8739 via Pixabay.com,

https://pixabay.com/en/chinese-medicine-donguibogam-2178253/

Page 93 Photo by user Maltz Evans via Pixabay.com,

https://www.flickr.com/photos/147974511@N04/35791448780/

References

Chinese Medicine - Travelchinaguide.com

https://www.travelchinaguide.com/intro/medicine.htm

Disease Patterns Within Traditional Chinese Medicine - Virtualchinesemedicine.com

http://www.virtualchinesemedicine.com/disease-patterns

Five Element Framework - Tcmworld.org

https://www.tcmworld.org/what-is-tcm/five-elements/

The Basic Content of the Five Elements Theory – TCMBasics.com

http://www.tcmbasics.com/basics_5elements.htm

The basics of traditional chinese medicine – AsktheScientists.com

https://askthescientists.com/traditional-chinese-medicine/

The Application of Yin Yang Theory in Traditional Chinese Medicine - Shen-nong.com

http://www.shen-nong.com/eng/principles/application1yinyang.html

Traditional Chinese Medicine – Wikipedia.org

https://en.wikipedia.org/wiki/Traditional_Chinese_medicine

Traditional Chinese Medicine – RennWellness.com

https://www.rennwellness.com/acupuncture/traditional-chinese-medicine-and-acupuncture.html

Traditional Chinese Medicine Benefits, Herbs & Therapies – Dr.Axe.com

https://draxe.com/traditional-chinese-medicine/

What Are Yin and Yang in Chinese Medicine? – AmCollege.edu

https://www.amcollege.edu/blog/what-are-yin-and-yang

What Is Qi? (and Other Concepts) – TakingCharge.csh.umn.edu

https://www.takingcharge.csh.umn.edu/explore-healing-practices/traditional-chinese-medicine/what-qi-and-other-concepts

What Is TCM? – TCMWorld.org

https://www.tcmworld.org/what-is-tcm/

Yin and Yang in Traditional Chinese Medicine - AmCollege.edu

https://www.amcollege.edu/blog/yin-and-yang-in-traditional-chinese-medicine

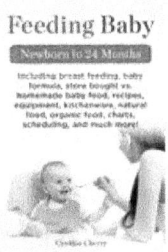

Feeding Baby
Cynthia Cherry
978-1941070000

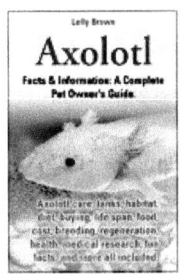

Axolotl
Lolly Brown
978-0989658430

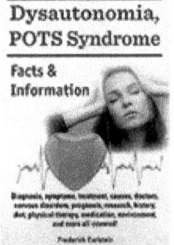

Dysautonomia, POTS Syndrome
Frederick Earlstein
978-0989658485

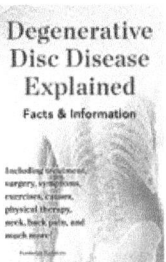

Degenerative Disc Disease Explained
Frederick Earlstein
978-0989658485

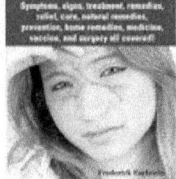

Sinusitis, Hay Fever,
Allergic Rhinitis Explained
Frederick Earlstein
978-1941070024

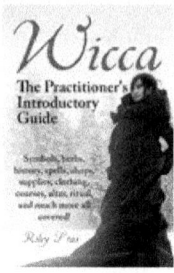

Wicca
Riley Star
978-1941070130

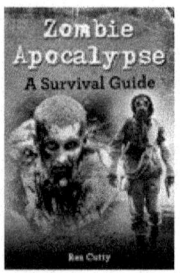

Zombie Apocalypse
Rex Cutty
978-1941070154

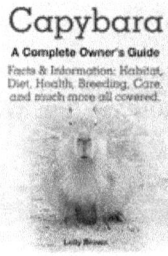

Capybara
Lolly Brown
978-1941070062

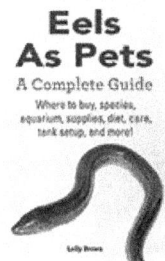

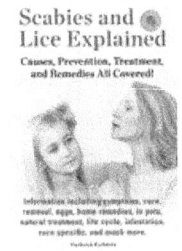

Eels As Pets
Lolly Brown
978-1941070167

Scabies and Lice Explained
Frederick Earlstein
978-1941070017

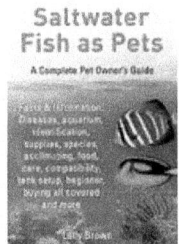

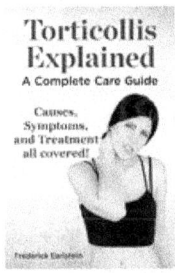

Saltwater Fish As Pets
Lolly Brown
978-0989658461

Torticollis Explained
Frederick Earlstein
978-1941070055

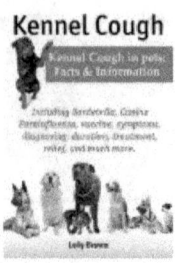

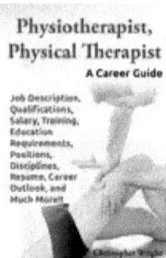

Kennel Cough
Lolly Brown
978-0989658409

Physiotherapist, Physical Therapist
Christopher Wright
978-0989658492

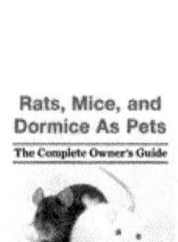

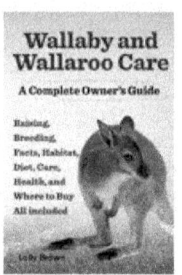

Rats, Mice, and Dormice As Pets
Lolly Brown
978-1941070079

Wallaby and Wallaroo Care
Lolly Brown
978-1941070031

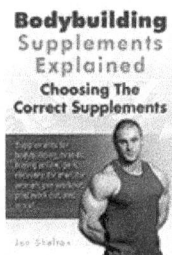

Bodybuilding Supplements
Explained
Jon Shelton
978-1941070239

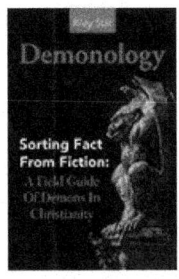

Demonology
Riley Star
978-19401070314

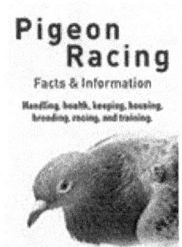

Pigeon Racing
Lolly Brown
978-1941070307

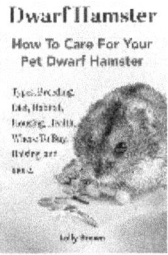

Dwarf Hamster
Lolly Brown
978-1941070390

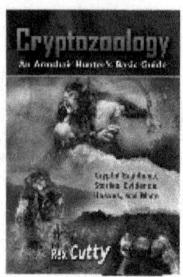

Cryptozoology
Rex Cutty
978-1941070406

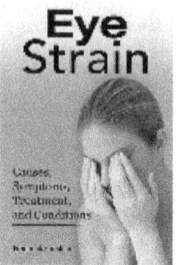

Eye Strain
Frederick Earlstein
978-1941070369

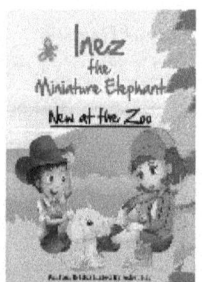

Inez The Miniature Elephant
Asher Ray
978-1941070353

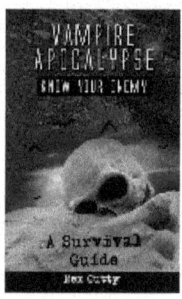

Vampire Apocalypse
Rex Cutty
978-1941070321

www.ingramcontent.com/pod-product-compliance
Lightning Source LLC
Chambersburg PA
CBHW060837050426
42453CB00008B/723